T0222177

FIELD GUIDE TO TELEHEALTH AND TELEMEDICINE FOR NURSE PRACTITIONERS AND OTHER HEALTHCARE PROVIDERS

Craig Sorkin, DNP, APN, RN, ANP-C, FNP-C, is an adult nurse practitioner who cares for patients at Riverside Medical Group (RMG) in Jersey City, New Jersey, and is RMGs first nurse practitioner. He received his master's degree with a focus in advanced clinical practice education at William Paterson University and his DNP at Drexel University. Dr. Sorkin is the current clinical lead of telemedicine at RMG and has been a driving force with telemedicine during the COVID-19 pandemic. In 2016, he coauthored *Adult-Gerontology and Family Nurse Practitioner: Self-Assessment and Exam Review.*

FIELD GUIDE TO TELEHEALTH AND TELEMEDICINE FOR NURSE PRACTITIONERS AND OTHER HEALTHCARE PROVIDERS

Craig Sorkin, DNP, APN, RN, ANP-C, FNP-C

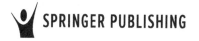 SPRINGER PUBLISHING

Copyright © 2022 Springer Publishing Company, LLC

Springer Publishing Company, LLC
11 West 42nd Street, New York, NY 10036
www.springerpub.com
connect.springerpub.com/

Acquisitions Editor: Rachel X. Landes
Compositor: Transforma

ISBN: 978-0-8261-7275-4
ebook ISBN: 978-0-8261-7292-1
DOI: 10.1891/9780826172921

21 22 23 24 / 5 4 3 2 1

The author and the publisher of this Work have made every effort to use sources believed to be reliable to provide information that is accurate and compatible with the standards generally accepted at the time of publication. Because medical science is continually advancing, our knowledge base continues to expand. Therefore, as new information becomes available, changes in procedures become necessary. We recommend that the reader always consult current research and specific institutional policies before performing any clinical procedure or delivering any medication. The author and publisher shall not be liable for any special, consequential, or exemplary damages resulting, in whole or in part, from the readers' use of, or reliance on, the information contained in this book. The publisher has no responsibility for the persistence or accuracy of URLs for external or third-party Internet websites referred to in this publication and does not guarantee that any content on such websites is, or will remain, accurate or appropriate.

Library of Congress Cataloging-in-Publication Data

Names: Sorkin, Craig, author.
Title: Field guide to telehealth and telemedicine for nurse practitioners
    and other healthcare providers / Craig Sorkin.
Description: New York : Springer Publishing Company, [2022] | Includes
    bibliographical references and index. | Summary: "Patients became
    responsible for monitoring their own blood pressures and glucose
    readings in a way they had never been responsible for previously.
    Patients who, under normal circumstances, would be admitted to the
    hospital without question were being discharged home, some even on
    oxygen or with bilateral pneumonia. How to manage a patient with mild
    hypoxemia from home when that patient cannot come to the office for
    periodic pulse oximetry monitoring? We found a smartphone application
    that offered pulse and pulse oximetry using their phone's camera"--
    Provided by publisher.
Identifiers: LCCN 2021041720 | ISBN 9780826172754 (paperback) | ISBN
    9780826172921 (ebook)
Subjects: MESH: Telemedicine | Mobile Applications | Nurse Practitioners
Classification: LCC R119.95 | NLM W 83.1 | DDC 610.285--dc23
LC record available at https://lccn.loc.gov/2021041720

CONTENTS

PREFACE

I have been interested in telemedicine and digital health since undergraduate nursing school. While other students were doing their medication math and pathophysiology research in bulky pocket guides, I was using my PalmPilot with great success. Fast-forward to graduate school, where I earned my adult nurse practitioner master's degree and family nurse practitioner postgraduate degree, and where I wrote several papers and completed presentations on the benefits and future of technology in medicine. My doctoral degree also had several reports and projects focusing on the topic. Never did I imagine how valuable technology would be to myself, my employer, and my patients.

I have been working on bringing telemedicine to my practice since 2015. After many ups and downs, it was finally brought to the front burner because of COVID-19. During this pandemic, years of research, long-winded meetings, and dedication paid off. We, like many other healthcare organizations, were thrust into a completely digital care plan when we had to vacate our brick-and-mortar locations. I was named the clinical lead of telemedicine at my practice and helped bring it to life.

The first day, I was the only provider with one assistant, and we saw 30 patients. The next day, we saw 60 patients with two assistants. By the end of the week, we had four providers and an entire team dedicated to this platform with more than 200 patients served in one day! The next week, as the crisis ramped up, we had more and more patients being seen digitally. After two months of the new normal during COVID-19, we had completed more than 100,000 telemedical visits across all our primary care and specialty care providers.

Patients became responsible for monitoring their own blood pressures and glucose readings. Patients who, under normal circumstances, would be admitted to the hospital without question were being discharged home, some even on oxygen or with bilateral pneumonia. How to manage a patient with mild hypoxemia from home when that patient cannot come to the office for periodic pulse oximetry monitoring? We found a smartphone application that offered pulse and pulse oximetry using their phone's camera. I have never prescribed more home monitoring equipment than during this period. Patients became their own nurses.

I hope you enjoy this book and are able to take some knowledge that has been hard-earned and battle-tested during one of the worst pandemics this society has ever seen. Digital health and telemedicine are here to stay. What remains to be seen is how far they will advance and how accepted they will become.

Craig Sorkin

I

TELEMEDICINE AND TELEHEALTH BASICS

TELEMEDICINE VERSUS TELEHEALTH

▥ Introduction

Telemedicine is one of the quickest growing fields inside of medicine. In one form or another, it has been around for generations. However, its popularity has skyrocketed and become a preferred source of seeking medical care. During the COVID-19 crisis throughout 2020, telemedicine was practically the only form of healthcare patients could receive outside of a hospital or drive-through clinic. Synchronized and asynchronized medical visits across the specialties, remote patient monitoring, and other forms of digital care have become a mainstay in the current healthcare climate.

What was once a "backup" form of healthcare suddenly was thrust onto the front burners. Practices were scrambling to stand up a digital platform and continue to care for their patients as well as continue a flow of revenue to keep their doors open. Digital health in all its formats was given special dispensations by the government, payors and organizations in order to help combat COVID.

Digital Health, Telemedicine, and Telehealth

The types of digital health available all allow for a certain factor of the care of the patient to be met. While the modalities may overlap, they each provide their own pros and cons. How they interact and lead to the final digital health platform will vary from practice to practice. While some may choose to only utilize one aspect, most will choose to use several. Software for personal use devices will continue to become more popular. There is a lot of ground to be covered in the future of these modalities.

Digital Health

Digital health is an umbrella term that incorporates telemedicine, telehealth, and remote patient monitoring. Under this umbrella, the medical services branched out and developed a new, modern modality to care for patients in a dynamic new manner.

Telemedicine

Telemedicine is the practice of medicine via a digital medium by a licensed practitioner. Medical visits completed using this medium allow for an assessment, diagnosis, treatment plans, and referrals to be initiated; an in-person evaluation can follow a telemedical visit. Depending on the state in which the provider is practicing, there may be limitations on the services that can be rendered and the manner in which they can be reimbursed. Certain states also require waivers to perform telemedical services.

This type of encounter can include evaluation and management of diagnostic tests such as laboratory evaluations, imaging results, and consultant reports. Telemedicine can be used for acute care illness and injury as well as monitoring chronic conditions. In situations in which care is being conducted for remote patients and patients who do not have specialized care available to them, telemedicine is an excellent modality to achieve some aspects of specialty care from the patient's home or local doctor's office. During the COVID-19 pandemic the rules and regulations directing telemedicine, especially with regard to Medicare patients, were significantly loosened. How these changes will proceed once the COVID pandemic is over is unknown.

Telehealth

Telehealth is the support services provided by a nonclinical provider, that is, nursing or medical assistance (electronic scheduling, etc.), and is usually seen as a supplement to telemedicine. Telehealth can also include medical education, administrative care, training events, and follow-up evaluations with nurses, dieticians, and physical and occupational therapists. Telehealth also incorporates the ability to provide medical education and offers an ability to provide in-service to providers and staff.

Examples of telehealth include the following:

- Nursing visits for close monitoring of new and chronic conditions

- Pharmacists offering advice about potential medication side effects and interactions

- Dieticians consulting about managing conditions utilizing the best approach to a patient's diet

Dieticians can ask patients to take the camera around their kitchen to show what the patient may think is healthy or demonstrate what type of food scale they use. A physical therapist (PT) or occupational therapist (OT) can see how a patient performs their activities of daily living. The PT or OT can also monitor the patient's gait and note any risks for fall or other factors of injury around the house. A pharmacist can see how a patient store and take their medication; for instance, are the medications organized or scattered? The pharmacist can also note if a patient is storing their medication correctly, for instance insulin stored out of the refrigerator. These services are traditionally nonreimbursable. However, during the COVID-19 pandemic there was a reduction in their restrictions that allowed these services to become reimbursable; this, however, varied from state to state.

Remote Patient Monitoring

Remote patient monitoring is the practice of allowing patients to monitor themselves while digitally transmitting that information to a provider or other members of the care team. While this is usually incorporated into telehealth services, it is fast becoming a field of its own. This section of the digital healthcare system allows for patients to be monitored in a condition most comfortable to them. Remote patient monitoring does not necessarily mean that patients or families must purchase new equipment, as most people have smartphones, smartwatches, and other pieces of hardware in their homes that can collect and transmit data to their providers. A multitude of applications on smartphones can monitor female health, track steps and workouts, and monitor dietary and medication compliance.

Remote patient monitoring seems to be among the last of the digital health buildup. This is most likely due to the need for extra equipment. However, the use of commercially available equipment such as smartwatches and other commercially available wearable technology has helped increase the popularity of this type of digital health. Application-based pulse oximeters proved to be an invaluable piece of technology during the beginning of the COVID-19 pandemic.

Overview of Challenges in Telemedicine

As an emerging form of care, telemedicine contains inherent challenges that are hard to overcome, such as clinical inability to do certain types of evaluations, billing concerns, and technological lack of proper infrastructure to complete an exam. Provider and patient hesitance to adopt a digital medical platform is also a factor. There are solutions in the works for all these concerns. However, legislation and business policies take time to change and become part of main care. Throughout 2020, it was clearly demonstrated that this new form of healthcare is dependable and available and that there is a niche for this type of service.

A confusing factor in telemedicine services is laws and regulations. These are controlled by federal, state, and institutional policies. Who can bill for services, who can prescribe, and what can be prescribed? Different states also have parity laws that determine if the insurance must pay for services rendered during a telemedical encounter. The COVID-19 pandemic changed a lot of the rules and regulations regarding digital health. Care between the states was allowed, Controlled Dangerous Substances (CDS) were allowed to be prescribed telephonically and electronically in states where this wasn't usually allowed. It seemed that there was a change to the regulations every time these data were solicited. Since the dust seems to have settled, the overall changes appear positive and embrace the usage of digital technology for healthcare needs.

Overview of Benefits of Telemedicine

The Centers for Disease Control and Prevention (CDC) offers the suggestion that telemedicine and telehealth will reduce healthcare costs and increase access to care, especially in underserved populations in rural areas (CDC, 2016). Telemedical visits in rural populations grew from 7,000 in 2004 to over 100,000 by 2013 (CDC, 2016).

Telehealth has grown greatly over the last 20 years. Mental health telemedicine alone has increased 45% over the last decade (Balestra, 2017). The CDC projects that state telemedicine and telehealth will be a $30 billion portion of healthcare.

The budding platform of telemedicine has the potential to improve communications not only between patients and providers but also among the providers and the interdisciplinary care team. The ability to provide medical education and share knowledge and techniques is also an important aspect of care (National Quality Forum, 2017).

Digital medicine has infiltrated every aspect of our lives. Smart devices check our heart rate, monitor an electrocardiogram, detect hydration level, monitor exercise patterns, and help women monitor menstruation and fertility. You can't help but see advertisements for telemedical services by large hospital chains and internet start-up companies on road signs, on social media, and in smartphone-application stores. Television commercials are dedicated to advertising the ease of obtaining "embarrassing" medications such as erectile dysfunction therapies, treatments for balding, and sexually transmitted disease monitoring.

Approaches to proper assessment techniques, visit etiquette, and how to assess your digital health approach are important aspects of digital health care. The ability to reach the masses and assess them in their comfort zone allows for the best quality care. Digital health also offers the benefits of being available on the timeline of the patient, and if the patient does not have insurance, this usually occurs at a lower price point.

There are many great resources to utilize during the discussion, implementation, and application of a digital health platform. The Center for Medicare and Medicaid Services, American Telemedicine Association, the CDC and the American Medical Association are just a few that offer great insights, documents, and playbooks to build and model platforms for success. The National Quality Forum also put forth a very succinct and practical guide for creating and supporting a digital health platform. The World Health Organization and the various academies of specialties and state board of medicine or nursing all offer opinions on the efficacy and need for digital health platforms. An organization must analyze the base information from these resources and formulate how to implement it in the organization. This is not an easy task, but to use the road already paved by others and build upon it eases the burden.

This book will hopefully answer questions on these topics and aims to enlighten emerging providers, administrators, and payors to the benefits of telemedicine and telehealth. With knowledge comes power and the ability to effect change. The future of telemedicine is in the hands of those who are rendering services. Technology can and always will catch up to the demand. The legislation and business need to be motivated to change. This will only come with continued proof that this method of practicing medicine is cost-effective with high patient and provider satisfaction.

History of Telemedicine

When the first telegraph was sent, we entered a new era in our society, one in which one side of the map could reach the other in a period of time previously unheard of. It was not long before healthcare providers used this ability for the medical needs of a population. Increases in the speed of care and the ability to obtain care from a distance all improve the overall health of society. What was telemedicine in times past is no longer considered such. However, the improvements and advancements that have occurred since have allowed this field of medicine to flourish.

Once more modern technology became available, the telephone was utilized to contact help, seek distant medical care, and increase the distance that one could reach the public. The ability to seek care over the telephone or summon a doctor without leaving the house had great advantages. In a time when most communities were served by a family doctor who performed all healthcare duties, having the ability to reach out to a specialist or get to a hospital when one or both could be hundreds of miles away could be the difference between life and death.

War has always unfortunately pushed technology and innovation forward. During World War II, medics and corpsmen on the frontlines used radio transmission to seek medical control from doctors stationed at headquarters. The wars in Korea and Vietnam sped up healthcare by increasing the availability of helicopter transport. The increased ability of medics and corpsmen to obtain direction and rapid medical evacuation from the battlefield has also proved to save a great many lives. Medical professionals on the front lines of battle could consult via radio and now with audio and video communications with a dedicated specialist to increase the survivability of our soldiers, sailors, marines, and airmen.

During the 1960s, space programs, based mostly in the USSR and the United States, had the ability to transmit the telemetry data of the astronauts (cosmonauts for the Soviets) back to home base. There was usually at least one physician on-site at mission control to monitor vital signs and assess any medical needs that could arise.

More recent history demonstrates a clear increase in the use of digital services. With the heightened performance of audio and video services via webcams, smartphones with front-facing cameras, and high-speed internet, digital health as we know it today is more widely available than ever. The last few years, with their corresponding increase in technology, have allowed the world of digital health to grow exponentially.

References

Balestra, M. (2017). *Telehealth and legal implications for nurse practitioners*, *14*(1), 33–39. https://doi.org/10.1016/j.nurpra.2017.10.003

Centers for Disease Control. (2020). *Telehealth and telemedicine.* https://www.cdc.gov/phlp/publications/topic/telehealth.html

National Quality Forum. (2017). NQF: *Telehealth framework to support measure development 2016–2017 - Description.* https://www.qualityforum.org/ProjectDescription.aspx?projectID=83231

TELEMEDICINE IMPLEMENTATION

Introduction

The first topic to cover is deciding what your practice's goals of digital health are. Once you decide your needs the market for the proper medium becomes the priority. There are many applications that utilize a computer or internet format versus an application-based platform versus a partition of the internal electronic medical record (EMR).

Questions to Ask Before Establishing a Digital Health Practice

- Is there a specific need?
- What are your state laws and billing practices?
- Do you want to provide a robust platform where you can offer more than audio and visual services (e.g., remote patient monitoring services)?
- The location of the service will also help determine the proper platform; will be primary location be an office setting?
- Or will it be an acute care or a skilled nursing facility (SNF)?
- Is the goal to be the patients' home?
- What is your target population?

The Implementation Team

Administration

The administration is responsible for overseeing all aspects of the digital health team. Usually they, in concert with the clinical team, choose which platform will be utilized, how it will be utilized, and the workflow. They have to train the managers and medical assistants on how to assist patients and providers when completing a telemedical evaluation. The administration team will usually work directly with the executive team or may be the conduit to the executive team.

The administration faces a unique challenge. They are often not the ones who are responsible for a specific platform's usage, but they are responsible for everything about it and often get the final vote on what products are used by the organization. The administrator must listen to clinical leadership and to their various department heads in order to initiate a successful and operation platform.

The administration's goals should include the following:

- A platform that is functional and liked by clinicians, staff, and patients
- A platform that is affordable
- Appropriate return on investment
- A platform that meets the needs of the practice

Clinical Leadership

The clinical leadership is responsible for determining how and when the digital health platform will be utilized. While it is up to individual providers to care for their patients, there can be protocols when certain medications should be utilized, when higher levels of care should be enacted, and when the visit is not appropriate for a telemedical platform. The clinical leaders should have the largest role in the selection of a platform or a vendor as they will be the most common users of said platform.

While clinical leaders are often senior clinicians, they may not be in the position to offer final approvals. The clinical leader must be well versed in billing and legal concerns as well as administrative functions such as revenue cycle and reimbursements. The clinical leader is the one who needs to know the material inside and out.

The clinical leaders' goals should include the following:

- A platform that is easy to use for all involved
- A platform that can be utilized to the highest level possible
- Inclusion of remote patient monitoring (RPM) technology (if desired)

Information Technologist

The information technologist (IT) will confirm that the current equipment, firewalls, internet bandwidth, and other technical features are at the minimal level to provide adequate and seamless services. The IT team is also responsible for the cybersecurity of the platform, staff, and providers as well as offering patients techniques on how to stay safe. An interruption in services leads to patients', providers' and auxiliary staff's dissatisfaction. It can lead to a catastrophic failure of the whole program.

The IT specialist will need to know the specific functions of the platform and their minimum requirements and assure that the hardware on both ends of the interaction can handle the need. While that is not a simple task for the clinical end, the IT specialist will have the ability to assure proper computers, tablets, or other electronic platforms. For the patient end, they will not be able to tell a patient to go out and buy a new computer. Rather, they should help the clinical leaders and administrators select a platform that is universal and is available for people with older computers, tablets, and smartphones so that they can still access it.

The IT's goals should include the following:

- A platform that doesn't exceed the current hardware of the organization
- A platform that doesn't require more infrastructure than the organization can support

Patient Advocates

Patient advocates should always be on the side of the patient while maintaining the ability of the provider to practice medicine. Patient advocates should assure that the platform and workflow will be patient-friendly. Patient advocates should also have a role in preparing literature for the patients on utilizing the platform once it is chosen as well as basic digital health success tips.

The patient advocate should know what the patient's previous complaints about service are and be ready to demonstrate from their perspective where a digital platform may fail. They should always be ready to play "devil's advocate" and try to find problems with the service before it even begins.

A patient advocate's goals should include the following:

- A platform that is easily accessible and understood by the patient
- A platform that doesn't require more technology than a patient would have available
- A platform that doesn't require the patient to call customer support for every usage

Billing and Coding Specialists

Billing and coding specialists assure the visits will be properly reimbursed. They should be up-to-date with what state and federal laws apply to their practice. Knowing which codes can and cannot be billed on telemedicine and what modifiers (if any) are required are key to knowing how to properly get paid. These specialists should also have knowledge of the appropriate waivers needed to perform these services, which clinicians can provide which type of services, and the settings from which the patient and clinician can complete a digital health assessment.

The billing and coding team is going to have one of the hardest jobs. They will need to know the current rules and regulations as well as any that may be changing. During the COVID-19 pandemic, there were several changes to the rules and regulations regarding digital health, especially with regard to government-based insurances (Medicare and Medicaid).

The billing and coding team's goals should include the following:

- A platform that tracks appropriate codes and modifiers
- Ease of use by the clinician and the billing and coding team

Legal Department

There should be a representative of the organization's legal department involved in the digital health process. While the majority of the aspects to care translate from a brick-and-mortar operation to a digital one, there are specific circumstances that require adjustments. Items such as consent forms, controlled substance prescriptions, and dealing with incapacitated adults or minors become difficult in the digital world.

Especially with the rapidly evolving changes that occurred during 2020 and into 2021, insurance companies, states, and the federal government were changing their telemedical rules and regulations on a monthly or even weekly basis.

The legal department should have the following goals:

- A platform that can assist with state-to-state rules (not allowing asynchronous visits in the states that prohibit)
- A reminder system for clinical staff for what can occur during a digital visit (this may not be a part of the platform as much as education surrounding the platform)

Platform Representative

The representative of the platform is required to assure that the platform is utilized to the highest ability it is designed to perform. There are usually many bells and whistles that can be unlocked inside of a platform, possibly at extra cost. The organization should know what is available and what the cost associated is prior to making final decisions. The organization should remember that the vendor's representative will likely be looking out for their interests. This is not to say that they will not be an advocate for the organization in question. However, keep in mind they are salespeople.

Their goal is simple: to SELL THE PLATFORM.

Appropriate Uses of Digital Platforms

Deciding if the complaint the patient is presenting for is appropriate for the digital platform is important for the successful completion of the telemedical or telehealth visit. While the provider cannot perform a physical exam via telemedicine, there are techniques that can be implemented using a family member or another trusted person. Later in this book we discuss means for self-evaluation and/or coaching family and friends through the physical exam. Special equipment can also be utilized to assist in the digital physical exam. While some visits may be considered "inappropriate" for digital health services, these patients may still benefit from a screening telemedical evaluation prior to an in-person, urgent-care, specialty-care, or emergency department visit being prompted (see Table 2.1).

Even for the "inappropriate" situations for telemedicine, there is a role for digital health. There is specific value for a clinician to lay eyes on a patient and gather further details. For chest pain, there are circumstances in which the emergency department is the only option. Other situations can be triaged out to a same-day specialist appointment or less urgent care. Not only does this allow for improved utilization management, but it also becomes a reimbursable interaction.

TABLE 2.1 **APPROPRIATE TYPES OF DIGITAL VISITS**

Appropriate	Inappropriate
Behavioral health (low risk)	Physical exams
Upper respiratory infections	First-time visits (state by state, CMS)
Urinary tract infections	Acute abdomen
Allergies	Chest pain in a high-risk category
	Comorbidities, high-risk family history
Rashes	Behavioral health (high risk such as suicidal)
Minor trauma—lacerations, abrasions, bites	
Lab and imaging reviews	
Follow-up after procedures	

CMS, Centers for Medicare and Medicaid Services.

Strategies for a Successful Transition to Digital Health

When offering digital health services, it is important to advertise and stress the impact and benefits of the new platform. The staff must know the appropriate and inappropriate types of encounters and the capabilities of digital health. Just as the front-desk staff plays a cheerleader role for the organization and the provider, they have the same responsibility for the telemedical and telehealth services. If the staff are cheerful and excited about the services, it will be popular. If they act as if they are baffled and troubled by it, patients will be scared and mistrustful of the digital solution.

The patient must be made aware of what would be required for an online evaluation. The type of technology (computer, tablet, phone with a camera) and the importance of a fast internet connection or high-speed cellular data connection all influence the quality of the digital health encounter. The patient should also be aware of the need to download specific software prior to the evaluation. Certain internet platforms only work on certain browsers. It is during the receptionist or call center interaction with the patient or, in some situations, a digital interaction that the patient must be made aware to alert for disability or language special requests. While the majority of office situations can accommodate for the common languages spoken in that area, the patient may still require translation. This includes patients that are hard of hearing and/or visually impaired as well as those who speak a different language than the provider and staff do. There will be circumstances in which the patient will need to be made aware that a digital interaction is not appropriate for them. This may dissipate in time; however, if the standard of care cannot be met for any reason, a digital encounter is not appropriate.

Where to Start

Similar to how clinicians are taught to assess a patient before making a diagnosis and creating a treatment plan, healthcare practices must conduct a detailed assessment of their current resources and goals before creating a telemedicine practice. This is a large-scale decision that could cost an organization significant money. Cautious decisions, planning, and preparatory work should go into all these initial steps and allow for the most successful outcome.

Recommendations of Best Practices

- Have a solid knowledge of the inner workings of the chosen platform.

- All users should know the normal functions; super-users, or practice champions, should have advanced knowledge.

- The practice's workflow should be implemented prior to going live.

- Establish a backup plan in case the primary option for digital health becomes unavailable.

- Implement appropriate protocols should emergent situations occur.

- Implement screening questions (COVID or other infectious disease–related).

- All records of digital health encounters should be kept as they would for in-person evaluations.

- Be consistent in updating the practice's knowledge of rules, regulations, and laws.

- Be aware of the current climate with telemedicine.

- Have staff properly assess who is interested in digital services versus who prefers in-person evaluations.

- Be conscientious when deciding upon a self-pay rate. It should balance the cost of covering services rendered while being affordable for the patient.

3

WORKFLOWS OF TELEMEDICINE

Introduction

Establishing a workflow for telemedical services is imperative for successful outcomes. Like building a pyramid, you must have a solid base to build up an effective program. Once the proper foundation is in place, a workflow for every aspect of the medical practice will help ensure the success of the program. It is imperative to understand the needs and desires of the program prior to initiating and planning everything surrounding it.

The American Medical Association (AMA) *Telehealth Implementation Playbook* identifies several steps to starting a digital health program at an organization.

Identifying a Need

Prior to the COVID-19 pandemic, telehealth was a budding field of medicine. During, and hopefully after, COVID-19, the field has grown exponentially. The federal and local governments as well as Centers for Medicare and Medicaid Services (CMS) changed many of the rules and regulations surrounding telemedical services, including eliminating the requirement that patients must be rural or remote and unable to obtain healthcare via another manner, the use of telephonic codes, and a multitude of others.

Identifying the target group is also important. While the CMS has started to allow for its customers to receive telemedical services, are those the patients who will be most served by this type of medical care?

Benefits of digital health include the following:

- Increases access to care
- Decreases costs
- Decrease exposure of potentially contagious disease
- Enables remote patients to seek care from centrally located specialists

Telemedicine can close care gaps, be used to make up missed appointments, and increase continuity of care. Telehealth allows for remote education and follow-up with patients and families. Remote patient monitoring allows for real-time supervision of a patient's metrics and allows for the ability for an immediate intervention to be put in place should a life-or-death situation present itself. Organizations must set realistic goals for their platforms and digital health departments. There are several concerns that should be identified and preliminary solutions formatted.

Concerns for the implementation team include the following:

- The scope of practice for the providers in the program
- How will the services be billed and reimbursed
- Who will oversee the implementation and maintenance of the software and hardware
- The overall budget
- Problems that can be solved by telemedicine
- Identification of care gaps that can be closed
- What patients can see via this platform
- Applicable laws, regulations, and statues

Budget

The budgetary constraints should be one of the first topics to be discussed after determining the need for digital health. Spending too much for a platform without demonstrating a way to recoup these funds and make a profit is a sure way to dissuade the leadership from proceeding with the program. The goal of the platform is to make everything smoother for the patient, which cannot happen if it does not become part of the organization.

Not everything needs to be the best and brightest when starting a program. Many practices start off with a basic electronic medical record (EMR) and an audio and video platform. From there, you can grow and scale as much as you can afford. There is always going to be another add-on that can be part of the system or another piece of remote patient monitoring; that does not mean it needs to be part of your program.

Forming the Team

The team for a digital health implementation must include leaders from administration, clinical fields, billing, and representatives of the various patient care areas (specialists, medical assistants, etc.).

Communication

Communication is key to the formation of the team. The leaders who compose the team bringing digital health to an organization should provide feedback throughout the implementation process. Their opinions must be valued and appreciated. They must be allowed to speak freely and offer pros and cons about the application of digital health. There should be team members from all areas of the organization with varied backgrounds so as to offer the broadest mindset to the goal of establishing a digital health platform.

Team members must be able to work together toward the common goal. Avoid duplicated roles among the team to decrease confusion. The team members should have clear roles and responsibilities, with each aspect of the building process assigned to one team or another. There needs to be coordination of the team to assure that there is focus and progress by the creation team toward meeting the goals of the organization.

■ Defining Success

This step allows for the establishment of the short- and long-term goals of the program. These goals must have measurable metrics to be properly evaluated by the teams.

Goals should include the following:

- Clear return of investment
- Clear fulfillment of the needs of the organization
- Clear benefit to the population served
- Clear benefit to the population served

Simple and measurable steps along the way will aid in defining success. There must be clear steps from the beginning all the way to a final product. How many of these steps are needed will depend on the nature of the organization, the scope of the project, bumps in the road, and how quickly solutions present themselves. A clear endpoint to establish when the product is ready for scaling throughout the organization is the final step in the implementation process.

The goals of the platform must align with the goals of the organization as well as the Quadruple Aim of healthcare:

- Improving the health of the population
- Enhancing the healthcare experience
- Reducing the cost of healthcare
- Improved clinical experience

Each organization will have its own aims and goals, but, for the most part, they are universal in healthcare. Focusing on healthcare outcomes, improving patient and clinician experiences, and decreasing the cost of healthcare will make the platform shine.

▓ Evaluating the Vendor

The implementation of a digital health platform must be completed as seamlessly as possible. The vendor of the platform is the sales team that is attempting to have a medical practice purchase their product. Some are stand-alone telemedical platforms, while some are integrated into the organization's EMR software. For a vendor and software to be successful, there must be the potential for a long-term relationship. The personalities must mesh, the flow of information must be without compromise, and the product must be affordable and practical. The company that supplies the software must be accessible to the leadership team and, throughout implementation, be available to patients, supportive staff, and clinicians. The success of the platform depends on its usability by patients and clinicians.

Essential vendor components to verify include the following:

- The quality of the company's software
- Business model
- Customer support
- Information technology (IT) support
- Ease of use

Software requirements include the following:

- Must be compatible with the current EMR
- Should provide a good workflow
- Must be secure with appropriate biometric security measure

    ☐   Informed consent for the practice must be adjusted to cover digital health services and protect against Health Insurance Portability and Accountability Act (HIPAA) violations.

The overall function of the platform must be evaluated, and the needs of the organization must be compared with the abilities of the software.

The parent company of the software platform should be evaluated for business practices, the cost of services and the cost of maintenance and upkeep.

While a medical practice is evaluating potential software companies, they must complete their due diligence and assure that the digital health vendors are successful and have not had severe customer service or technological problems in the past.

While each medical practice has different needs and expected outcomes from a vendor, the past records of a vendor should serve as a baseline for its functionality and ability to provide a practical, profitable, and functional platform.

Any fees should be transparent and made available. The vendor should also be able to prove that its platform can function for the population it is being purchased for.

Certain platforms are more geared toward certain populations, specialties, and usages. This must be considered when purchasing said platform. While being specific can be good, it may be better to purchase a more generalizable digital health platform. The vendor must be able to serve the clinicians, dieticians, therapists, nursing, administrative, IT, and all other users equally and productively. There should not be difficulty in any aspect of the platform.

Difficulties of the platform may include the following:

- IT glitches
- Poor customer service
- Technological needs that exceed what the general-use population will have

- Technological needs that exceed what the organization will have

- Non-user-friendly interfaces

The software platform should be easily accessible for all parties and be amenable to include any remote patient monitoring services that the practice wishes to implement.

The leadership team of the organization must utilize their own instincts, supportive materials, and factual data when validating a vendor company. There should not be a blind selection process or one that is focused on money. If the platform does not meet expectations, both patients and the provider will be dissatisfied. This will lead to overall dissatisfaction with the digital health application for the practice.

▓ Making the Case and the Project Proposal

The final approval for the selection and implementation of a digital health platform at an organization must come from the executive leadership. The executive team should take information, data, and suggestions from their project leaders but complete their own verification of all prior to their decision.

The project lead team should have clear-cut information about all steps previously discussed. They should know the initial costs, maintenance costs, projected financial gains, and benefits for patients and the staff. The selection of the vendor being brought before the executive team should be clear, concise and have all the relevant information. The creation team should be able to anticipate questions and concerns of the executive team when crafting the project proposal.

Requirements for the project proposal include the following:

- What resources would be needed from the organization and from the vendor

- An estimated budget

■ The value it will bring to the organization

■ The security and infrastructure changes that will be required.

A leader of each section of the project team should be present to bring up how each department will benefit from the digital health solution. There will be a give-and-take to the selection process as there is likely not going to be a 100% perfect answer. The pros should always out weight the cons of the vendor and the software.

■ Contracting

Signing a contract requires careful steps to assure both sides will mutually profit.

Steps include the following:

■ Reviewing the contract

■ Negotiating to the mutual benefit of both parties

■ Legal review

■ Signatures and execution of the contract

Both sides must be assured they can meet expected goals, timelines, and budgetary constraints. Prior to signing any legal documents, the organizational power structure must be of one mind without any concerns as to the quality of the product or any other issue. The contract must specifically name the resources available, support, and how to grade success. Timelines must be specific, attainable, and assure satisfaction on both sides. Legal representatives from both sides should be able to adjust the contract as needed to assure that both sides will get what they signed on for.

The supply line of the hardware and other materials should be part of the contract negotiations. The contract should clarify quality control and monitoring of the equipment for damage and returns to the organization. If the items are damaged or lost who is responsible? It will be important to know if the organization is responsible for any costs associated with damaged or lost equipment.

This step assures both sides will get what they want out of the deal. It can also break the deal if the vendor and the organization cannot come to an agreement on certain steps, metrics, goals, costs, and support structure. This step should also include what happens if a problem occurs and when the contract can be broken (terms of terminating contract, cost of terminating).

■ Designing the Workflow

The workflow should be tested for the functionality of the platform and role adjustments. Who will be responsible for which tasks and where they will physically be (in office, home, other location) all need to be assessed. Who will complete which aspects of care, maintain scheduling, complete intake, conduct assessments, process billing, and all sections of the continual project team will be important.

The clinical staff—medical assistants, nurses, providers, and especially the support staff—should all know how to utilize the platform. The support staff will be responsible for coaching patients through downloading or accessing the platform to assure a seamless flow of care during a telemedical or telehealth assessment. In addition to verbally instructing patients, they can use educational materials, pamphlets, emails, and other means of getting this information to patients created for this purpose. All staff should be able to properly upload or send data from a remote patient monitoring device. Scheduling staff should know how to assess if a patient's complaint is appropriate for telemedical services.

Advertising the new platform will be part of the workflow as well. The public relations department or whoever is responsible for social media at the organization and the administration should make a large public push for advertising the new service. This push should be made in steps, first, by advertising the pending implementation of the platform and, second, by announcing the digital health service going live.

Preparing the Care Team Prior to Go-Live Date

Leadership should assess the clinical staff for ability and desirability to function as an online medical provider. The best outcome of clinical metrics for digital health comes when the clinician, support staff, and patients are all exciting and well informed about digital health.

There should be an informal information-gathering session that assesses who among the clinicians, support staff, and others at the organization is interested in working with the digital health team. Passion and a full understanding of the services to be provided will go a long way in creating and operating a digital health care team.

Proper protocols about treatment plans and emergency situations and any other clinical pearls should be addressed prior to opening the platform to the public. Test runs with clinicians and staff should be completed to assure seamless functionality of the platform and assure the staff are aware of the workflow. Moving forward, routine updating of clinical protocols, system updates, and check-ins by the vendor, support staff, and clinical leaders will assure proper use of the platform.

First, staff and clinical leaders should be trained by the vendor's training staff. Once certain in their abilities, they can train other staff and clinical members. These members become the practice's superusers or practice champions. These practice champions should remain available to the clinical leaders and auxiliary staff should the need occur, especially in the beginning. Also responsible for patient education, they should teach patients and their families how to properly set up their personal machines for digital healthcare.

Practice billing and legal officials should update their knowledge base about billing codes and other policies regarding telemedicine, telehealth, and remote patient monitoring services on a regular basis. Especially since March 2020, there have been significant changes in the world of digital health and telemedicine. What once was completely nonreimbursable is not a practice norm. What rules and regulations at the state and federal levels will remain post-COVID is to be determined. It is my personal belief that the majority of the changes that have occurred, especially those regarding billing and location practices, will remain. The interstate care and some of the other very liberal changes will most likely revert to a more conservative way of practice.

IT professionals from the vendor and the organization should assure that all hardware and software are ready to perform their required duties. Cybersecurity measures should be updated, and proper electronic ports should be opened to allow terminals to get safely around the firewalls most organizations will have in place.

Throughout the process, there should be proper feedback to clinical and administrative leaders about how all aspects of the virtual platform are functioning. Clear roles and responsibilities should be defined to avoid confusion, duplicating tasks and avoid missteps by staff members.

Partnering With the Patient

The success of digital health depends upon the satisfaction of the patient. If patients are not happy with any aspect of care (platform accessibility and usability, satisfaction with the provider, satisfaction with the auxiliary staff, and anything else with the telemedical or telehealth visit) the platform will fail. Education packets that can be sent to the patients may aid in the success of the platform. This allows the patients to feel in control of the situation and should increase satisfaction.

Subjects for education packets may include:

- When to use telemedicine
- How to access the platform
- What software may need to be downloaded
- If any insurances are excluded

When remote patient monitoring, patients must have access to all products needed for the devices (batteries, test strips, etc.). Telephone triage of previously established protocols should be addressed with patients as early on as possible to avoid frustration.

Reminder services such as emails or text messages through the practice's EMR, the digital health platform, or from the practice's auxiliary staff can prevent no-shows, late visits, or other complications. Parents should be reminded that they will need to be present for a minor child and that the child must be present during the visit, not sleeping or otherwise occupied. The patient or family can also be made aware of translation services available. Similar to when providing in-person care, support staff should make sure patients stay as close to their scheduled appointment as possible.

Some organizations may choose a "Uber" approach, that being clicking a button on a smart device and connecting to a provider. This technique offers the added benefit of being available to a patient's needs but requires the organization to have a provider ready for these calls and not otherwise occupied with in-person visits or other tasks.

■ Implementing

Practice runs prior to the final implementation of the product should be utilized.

The following topics can be included in a practice run:

- Proper scheduling techniques
- Overlapping visits and management thereof
- Enactment of emergency protocols (chest pain, etc.)

Practice scenarios should be plotted out starting with scheduling and building to the first patient contact all the way through the provider interaction with the patient, follow-up care, and further appointment scheduling. The administration should take the time to properly format the scenario to stress areas of concern, areas of known weakness, or areas where danger to the patient may occur, such as:

- Nonappropriate care rendered digitally
- Missed follow-up appointments

Tracking successful metrics is an important aspect of this care. Auxiliary staff should ramp up the focus on digital health. Everyone in the organization should be ready to support patients and staff. The IT team should be ready to support clinicians and patients. The first few days should include the close monitoring or workflow; patient, staff, and clinician satisfaction; and, over the first billing cycles, how revenue is received (copays, insurance payments).

The need to evaluate if malpractice coverage will cover digital health and telemedical services is important when implementing these into an organization. Most insurance companies will include digital practice in their policies while others require adding a rider to cover these services.

Evaluating Success

When evaluating success, use previously established metrics to measure. These will vary slightly practice-to-practice but will overall involve patient and provider satisfaction, the functionality of the program, the revenue collected for services rendered, and the overall health of the population serviced.

If metrics are not met, a process to evaluate why must be instituted. Clinical and administrative leaders must utilize verbal, written, and other forms of feedback (patient satisfaction surveys) to update and modify workflows. If the problem pertains to the vendor or software, the proper customer support from their end should be evaluated. The contract should have terms of when and how it can be broken if needed.

■ Scaling

To expand the software platform from a trial period to practice-wide can only be completed after meeting the initial metrics. The clear, concise goals that were established before this process started must be met, and all involved parties must be satisfied.

The workflow put into place during the initial test phase should be reevaluated for its application for the entire practice. Adjustments will need to be made for specialist care, remote patient monitoring, and other aspects that may or may not have been included in the initial test phase.

Any problems, concerns, or questions should be answered or addressed prior to scaling the application. The program's idiosyncrasies and the manner in which they can be quickly and simply overcome should be addressed.

The ability to market to new patients and new providers and to make the program a bigger success also becomes applicable during this step. Also, during this step there can be strides made in marketing the new platform to local businesses, schools, and colleges in an effort to expand the client base of the organization.

A workflow for day-to-day practice utilizing the digital health platform can be broken down into before the visit, the visit and after the visit.

▩ Before the Visit

Before the visit, the patient must be provided appropriate information about the visit, limitations of the abilities of telemedicine or telehealth, and what the visit will entail. For new patients, they must have their insurance verified and copay or deductible collected.

Patients must know how to access the digital health platform and when to join the room for the meeting. A triage process should be implemented at this stage to assure that the visit is appropriate for telemedical services. There is always the chance that a person's request for telemedicine service is inappropriate (physical exams, high-risk complaints).

▩ The Visit

For the visit to occur, the patients must go through a virtual check-in process prior to being evaluated by the clinician. The flow of data collection varies organization to organization and department to department.

Medical assistants should collect data from patients during the time there are in the digital waiting room. Information such as medical, surgical, and medication history and allergies, as well as any other information, could be adjusted. Any vital signs that could be collected by the patient at home with remote patient monitoring equipment should be gathered and placed into the patient's medical records. The medical records should be reviewed by the provider as well. In many states, this is a requirement for telemedical services. If the patient is located in the primary care provider's (PCP) office and the telemedical service is with a specialist, the provider and staff of the PCP should be able to complete vital signs, EKG, and point-of-care (POC) testing to aid the specialist is management and treatment.

The virtual exam room should be calm and reassuring. Both sides should have a calm, quiet room in which to complete the evaluation. The provider should complete the evaluation in a calm, collected, and reassuring manner.

▤ After the Visit

After the visit, the patient must be able to obtain their prescriptions, blood work, imaging, or any other medical intervention that may be ordered during the evaluation. The checkout staff member can arrange proper follow-up care and assure patients have appointments with their PCP and any appropriate specialist.

This phase can also include assessments of satisfaction from patients and providers about the platform and digital health as a whole (see Appendix D for a sample patient satisfaction survey). The after-visit phase also includes the coding and billing of a visit as well as assessing and potentially reevaluting reimbursement for the services rendered.

Having a well-thought-out workflow and assuring that staff and providers are all aware of their respective roles and responsibilities will make the integration of a digital platform that much smoother. There will always be bumps along the way that need to be sorted out, but proper planning can prevent these from becoming serious and possibly jeopardizing the digital health platform. Negotiations with the vendor and discussions with the leadership and executive teams of the organization will assure that everyone knows what they are getting from each section of the team.

4

TELEMEDICINE PLATFORMS, FORMATS, AND LOCATIONS

▧ Telemedicine Platforms

There are many platforms available to perform telemedical services. They all come with benefits and demerits. They range from those included in electronic medical records (EMRs) to white-label products designed to fit all a practice's needs.

The most popular platforms are usually the most user-friendly ones. There is no benefit to having a digital health solution if your patients and staff cannot utilize it. If it takes your auxiliary personnel precious time to explain over and over again how to access the platform and communicate with the provider, you lose time, productivity, and money. The platforms included within an EMR are usually less expensive while the white-glove options, the platforms that are designed specifically for an organization are usually the most expensive.

How to Select a Platform

When selecting a platform, assuring that the platform is safe and secure with adequate customer service for both the patients and providers is extremely important. The business model of the platform being considered is important as well:

- Is the business successful?
- Is the business publicly traded?

- If the business is not able to make money for itself, is it doing something wrong?

- Is there a problem with its platform?

The vendor of the platform should be open and honest about any and all problems associated with its software or business and any interventions it has planned to remedy these concerns. The more upfront and honest a company is, the more likely there will be a successful relationship. While this is true about anything, this field being so new requires an extra level of caution upon forming relationships.

Customer Service

The customer service of the platform provider must be able and willing to answer any inquiries at any time requested. If a patient or provider is unable to get the technical help that is required to make the platform successful, it will not be. While the organization is responsible for the hardware (computers, tablets, wireless or wired internet connection) the platform is responsible for the software.

The User Interface

The most important aspect of the platform is the user interface. If providers, patients, and staff all have difficulty accessing and utilizing the software, it will not integrate successfully. A simple but secure login, easy interaction with the digital health provider, and a simple disconnect make the process smooth and enjoyable. Platforms that offer integrated monitoring services and the ability to see patient images (digital stethoscopes, EKGs, ENT exams, etc.) all are nice, but if they are not easily accessible, most patients will not even make it that far to enjoy these perks.

Cybersecurity

Evaluating how the platform is secured and protected is a primary concern in selecting a platform. If the platform is protected by passwords or biometrics, this may play a role in usability. How the patient, clinicians, and staff access the program is another area of concern. Overly cumbersome security is not user-friendly. On the other end, having a platform without adequate security is a problem of a different sort. The information technology (IT) professionals should evaluate the level of encryption built into the software and the primary hardware it will use.

For some platforms, the vendor and itsrepresentatives can see clinical information rather than just itsown software data. If the proper nondisclosure agreements are in place, proprietary information will remain confidential. Organizations can also require vendors to sign Health Insurance Portability and Accountability Act (HIPAA) documents for additional security.

All technology assumed from outside vendors must be assessed for their cybersecurity protocols:

- Are they utilizing up-to-date security protocols?
- Is the encryption at or above industry standards?
- Have they had security breaches previously?
- If they have, what did they do to counter them?
- Do they employ "white hat" hackers to test their system?

The ability of the remote patient monitoring technology to interface with the software digital health platform and electronic medical record is another concern.

- Is there an automatic bridge?
- Does a bridge need to be created or developed?
- What is the cost for this integration?
- What is the software and hardware demands for it?

The security of data transfers and any weblinks is an important factor in selecting a platform. While the provider may be logged into a terminal in a secure office with biometric assess, secured connections, and two-step logins, that may not be true for patients. Patients will most likely be logging in from a personal device and may also be on an unsecured network (restaurants, library, college campus, etc.). The platform should be able to speak clearly as to how personal information from these unsecured locations will be protected.

The security of the digital health program is important for success, safety, of HIPAA information and the protection of the integrity placed upon us as healthcare providers. By law, medical providers are held responsible for maintaining the security of HIPAA-inclusive information. This includes, but is not limited to, name, date of birth, diagnosis, medical and surgical history, treatment plans, and results of laboratory and imaging. Working with IT professionals both inside an organization and with the vendor is key to maintaining the security of the digital health assessment.

Patients can protect their security in many ways. They can conduct their assessments in a private location, away from others to protect their data. If they must complete their evaluation in a public location, headphones can be utilized to decrease audio interference and to maintain HIPAA; this, however, does not stop others from hearing their voices, only the providers. The patient should also be instructed in the pre-visit period how to assure a secure connection to the platform. This is usually under the care of the vendor's software; however, the patient may need to adjust internet settings for themselves to keep their privacy.

Security risks have been linked to approximately 80% of all providers completing digital health evaluations (Filkins et al., 2016). Patients and staff should be instructed to not open links or emails that do not appear to be appropriate, come from unknown sources or promise services that are not likely to be available. During the COVID-19 pandemic when Zoom was becoming more popular, there was initially concern with the security of their chat pages as information there was apparently accessible and if included private information could be stolen.

The vendor's software and remote patient monitoring (RPM) hardware usually include exceptional security metrics. These will include, but are not limited to, password protection, biometric accessibility, two-step verifications, and other measures to assure that only the patient can access their portal. The same is true for the staff and providers, especially the providers with prescriptive capabilities.

Security breaches not only lead to problems with HIPAA compliance, the loss of proprietary information, and the embarrassment of the patient and the provider but can also be associated with heavy fines and civil or criminal litigation. The security of the entire computer system of an organization could be corrupted by one link in an email. If this breach becomes public, revenue could be lost not only to fines, legal fees, and the cost of finding and fixing the problem but also in the loss of current and future patients.

When RPM is being utilized for the patient evaluation, the devices in question must have been approved for use by the Food and Drug Administration. This demonstrates that these devices have been screened for cyberattack risks. While this seems to be from a bad spy movie, there is always the potential that a patient's medical device could be hacked and provide false data to the provider, be programmed to harm the patient, or other means of interfering with the flow of lifesaving information.

All devices utilized for the digital health platform by an organization should have all virtual entry and exit ports secured. There should be no ability for the user to install or remove data to the device (except for the approved system administrators). All software on the devices, either digital health–related or not, should be secured and verified prior to being installed, upgraded, or otherwise maintained. Proper security login procedures should be in place to assure that the person signing in is the one that should be accessing that material. Workstations should maintain HIPAA compliance by not being visible to nonclinical staff and be properly secured when that person leaves their terminal.

Security is vital to the success of an organization. No one wants to be the source of a breach due to a lack of focus or breach of protocols. Most organizations have these procedures in place to discuss during the onboarding of new providers and staff. However, the introduction of new platforms needs to be informed by any and all ways to protect themselves, their patients, the organization, and all data transferring back and forth.

■ Telemedicine Formats

There are many methods to preforming successful telemedical services. These are often decided upon by patient needs, state and federal laws, and practice workflow.

The most common techniques include:

- Real-time interactive
- Store and forward
- Remote monitoring

Real-Time Interactive

Real-time interactive, otherwise known as synchronous, is the most common format of telemedical service. A patient and a provider meet in a digital patient care setting for the purpose of providing healthcare. This platform integrates the most information with the highest level of care. Instruments such as RPM can be integrated into this platform, allowing not only a visual and patient-assisted physical exam but a real-time exam of body systems not usually assessable over digital means as well. Acute interventions and the management of urgent and emergent situations are best dealt with on a real-time interactive platform. Real-time interactive care allows for the patient and the provider to have immediate satisfaction and offers the ability to perform the highest quality of care. This is the format most likely paid for by all the payors including Medicare and Medicaid. This format also allows metrics such as hierarchical condition category coding, care gaps, and others that are required to be addressed by Centers for Medicare and Medicaid Services and some private payors.

Store and Forward

Otherwise known as asynchronous, this format is used when a patient will record images or video and forward it to the provider for future assessment. This allows the patient to store an audio and video message and send it to the provider to review at a future time. This is an exceptionally convenient option. However, a vast number of states and insurance companies do not reimburse for this type of telemedical service. This format loses the ability to act in a time-sensitive matter. In states that allow this type of telemedical care, the staff setting up the visits should inform patients that anything of an urgent, emergent, or time-sensitive nature should not be addressed utilizing this platform.

Remote Monitoring

Remote monitoring is used when devices are left with the patient or in a central location that is easily assessable. Blood pressure cuffs, glucometers, thermometers, scales, and several other devices are used to record patient data that are forwarded to the provider. This can occur in real time or in a bundle to be provided to the care team on a daily, weekly, monthly, or quarterly schedule.

RPM incorporates durable medical equipment into the digital world. This equipment may fall into the real-time arena (digital stethoscopes, EKGs, ENT scopes) or store and forward (recording and sending blood pressures, glucose readings, pulse oximetry, etc.). The utilization of an RPM can be integral to the patient's well-being. The ability to have the clinician monitor the patient's vital signs, glucose, or other healthcare data in real time or on a set schedule allows for care to not go every 3 months until the next visit but rather be completed in a period prior to an injury to the patient. This not only keeps the patient safe but also allows for decreased hospitalizations and decreased likelihood of comorbidities occurring.

Choosing a Telemedicine Format

The format a practice will choosefor digital health services will likely depend on state and federal laws surrounding the services as well as the regulations put forth by government and commercial payors. In states where all options are covered and reimbursable, the provider and the patient can choose which is best based upon the situation. Certain medical evaluations cannot meet the standard of care (the key phrase in providing safe and effective telemedical services) without being conducted in real time. While store and forward offers convenience, it may not prove to be effective for a specific complaint. An RPM may be utilized alone or in conjuncture with one of the other formats. How the organization uses these services will be as varied as the practices themselves.

▨ Locations of Telemedicine

The ability to reach our patients is paramount. A specialist in a major city can aid in the care of a patient in the most remote location. Major events, such as blizzards, hurricanes, and, most recently, COVID-19, do not have to degrade the care provided to patients at home and in the hospital. The provider caring for a range of patients does not have to leave their office or home to assess a patient in a faraway nursing care facility or an acute care facility. These are all small examples of how this world of digital medicine can benefit the masses.

Inpatient and rehab facility care offers a unique application for digital health and telemedicine. While the majority of care will be rendered face-to-face, there are opportunities to implement telemedicine in the interest of patients and providers. Teleneurology and cardiology should come to the front of one's mind. The ability to have a neurologist offer an opinion about a patient who may be having a stroke or a cardiologist for a patient having a potential heart attack can save heart and brain tissue. These teleservices are especially important in a facility without the availability of surgical intervention as they can speed up the process of getting the patient transferred to an appropriate care facility.

Patients receiving these telemedical specialty services from home or from the primary care provider's office can avoid unnecessary emergency department visits or be sent directly to an appropriate care facility (one that has the interventional services they may require) instead of wasting time at an inappropriate facility. Telepsychiatry can also intervene and offer the patient a place to be cared for other than the emergency department's crisis unit. However, proper care always dictates the telemedical role. If the patient is not in an appropriate facility and an emergency arises, the clinician should revert to what protocols are in place prior to the implementation of digital health services.

The usage of telemedical services from a school or office building location can help maintain a healthy school system and workforce. The ability to keep workers working should the need for simple care (lab results, refills, chronic care follow-ups) can be done on the lunch hour. People may not have to leave for unnecessary reasons, and a qualified medical practitioner can decide if a person is safe to stay at school or work. For children, the telemedical services could allow a clinician to evaluate a patient remotely given that the school has proper consent and equipment available. This would allow the child to be evaluated and managed without waiting for a parent to leave work to come and take the child to the provider's office. Again, safety and medical appropriateness for these situations will vary contracts as well in place for these services and patient or parental consent.

The location of digital health services will depend on many factors. State legislation regarding telemedical services, protocols in place for an organization, and contracts in place for which telemedical services will be used at a particular facility are just a few factors. Overall, the digital world is meant to be used in remote and distant locations, and care should benefit from its availability. Assuring that the patient stays safe is the primary goal of care, and should a situation arise in which digital health cannot meet the needs of the patient, the provider and care organization should revert to their backup protocols.

▪ Reference

Filkins, B. L., Kim, J. Y., Roberts, B., Armstrong, W., Miller, M. A., Hultner, M. L., Castillo, A. P., Ducom, J. C., Topol, E. J., & Steinhubl, S. R. (2016). Privacy and security in the era of digital health: What should translational researchers know and do about it? *American journal of translational research, 8*(3), 1560–1580.

5

LIMITATIONS AND RESTRICTIONS OF TELEMEDICINE

Introduction

All digital services must be at the same level as if the provider, auxiliary staff, or educator were in the same room as the patient or population they serve. The law mandates that the standard of care must be met. For example, any service rendered digitally should be at the same level of care as in-person. Digital health has come a long way in a relatively short time. However, technology must keep up with the demands and resources available. The standards we are held to must remain high. There is still the need to maintain a standard of care in the digital services we provide. While the vast majority of services can be rendered digitally, the care provider must use their judgment to know when to refer the patient to an in-person evaluation.

Availability of Technology

For Individuals

Patients must be able to access and utilize the services to enjoy the benefits of digital health. They must have an appropriate smart device—a tablet, a smartphone, a computer with camera and microphone—as well as a service—cellular or internet—to utilize the digital health platform.

In this day and age, it is very unlikely to come across a person of the 18–64 demographic without a smart device; however, it is not a given that patients will have access to the minimum service requirements.

For Organizations

The available technology at an organization is another limiting factor. There has to be a sufficient supply line for the products that an organization wishes to institute. How the provider practices and if it is being completed in a safe and effective manner can lead to concerns with the quality of digital health. When attempting to utilize remote patient monitoring, the patient and the provider must be able to access the hardware and software to perform these tasks.

For Countries

While telemedicine and digital health are a common occurrence in the United States, other countries may lack the infrastructure required to support a digital health approach. There are products and companies that exist with the technology to serve third-world countries with digital health solutions. Offer packages include remote laboratories, monitoring technology, and the ability to transmit the data to a major medical center. However, this is not the norm; it is the exception.

Future governmental or nongovernment organizations could continue this trend and produce care packages specifically for supplying and maintaining remote monitoring and telemedical services to remote areas of the globe. This is not a short-term solution by any means. It will require significant infrastructure and financing.

Just think about how many lives could be saved if there was the ability to offer remote care services to villages, towns, and cities that otherwise depend on one or two under-supplied medical providers. In essence, they could become force multipliers with the ability to train members of the community on the application of the devices and then monitor them from a distant location. Not only would the care quality increase, but the safety of the medical professionals in the more turbulent areas of the globe and the ability to incorporate more sophisticated techniques also become possibilities.

Human Error

As remote patient monitoring becomes more popular, the limitation of a patient's ability to follow instructions must be taken into account. The patient must be able to perform tasks as directed when they are directed to do so. The patient and their family will act as the hands of the provider, and the provider should remain cognizant of their level of abilities.

This is the area in which an organization's support staff should shine. They should know the product inside and out and be able to effectively walk patients and their families through the application and usage of the individual devices. The support staff of an organization essentially becomes the first-line information technology (IT) support as they are usually more known to patients and their families than the support help line of the supplying company.

Digital Concerns

Digital concerns are also a limitation to proper and complete telemedical services. There is always the chance that technological problems and security breaches lower the quality of digital health services (Balestra, 2017). If security does not allow for easy access to the service, both parties will be frustrated. However, too lax security risks breaches. This is a very fine line to walk, but most digital health platforms can do so successfully.

▓ State Restrictions

State lines also pose a limitation to digital health services. Usually, patients and providers reside in the same state, but occasionally patients may seek services while out of state. The rule of telemedical visits is that the provider must hold a license in the state that the patient resides in. The only exception is if the patient is an established patient and is visiting outside of their permanent state of residence. Depending on the state of practice, guidelines for care across state lines vary. The nurse (or physician) license compact is a legislative body working to create an interstate licensure process. See the table in the providers and laws chapter about this across state lines licensure information.

Prescribing medications can also be affected by state law. Some states put forth legislation that pharmaceuticals and therapies can only be prescribed after an in-person evaluation. In this case, a digital platform would be more useful for follow-up care than to establish new patients. Other states limit the prescription of controlled substances, or certain categories of Controlled Dangerous Substances, constraining the ability to provide postoperative care or drug rehabilitation care that requires medications such as methadone or suboxone. States and payors may also allow only certain diagnoses for new versus established patients. The Centers for Medicare and Medicaid Services and individual state practice acts are probably the best resources to guide an organization for this limitation.

HIPAA Compliance

The Health Insurance Portability and Accountability Act (HIPAA) laws must be strictly maintained during a telemedical evaluation. This can prove to be a challenge as a big draw of remote services comes from being able to see a provider wherever and whenever. This can include public places, that is, trains, stores and so forth. The provider must be vigilant that HIPAA material, such as diagnosis, treatment plans, and medical history, remains confidential during these encounters. Patients must be coached on how to protect their HIPAA material.

Navigating Limitations

Limitations and restrictions are a part of life. How an organization and the medical community as a whole overcome these will make digital health more mainstream. Inconsistencies with payor/payee relationships can lead to barriers in an effective digital health implementation. If state law dictates limitations on what can be prescribed during a digital health assessment, there will be a lack of confidence and more restrictions on who can complete a telemedical visit. What types of visits, who can bill, how much reimbursement is to be paid, and if copayments will be collected all vary state to state. These are just some of the limiting factors, and as the service becomes more popular, certainly more will appear. Time will allow for some of these issues to be corrected, but there will always be limits and restrictions.

There must also be provisions made to remain compliant with the Americans with Disabilities Act. There must be an ability to provide these services for patients who are hard of hearing, vis impaired, or do not speak the language. Many software platforms come with the ability to auto-translate dialogue. If it gets to a point where the patient cannot safely or effectively use the software or hardware, they should be directed back to the default brick-and-mortar care solution. Utilizing these services should not pose unnecessary risks to the patients we serve.

Reference

Balestra, M. (2017, December 11). *Telehealth and Legal Implications for nurse practitioners.* https://www.npjournal.org/article/S1555-4155(17)30808-5/fulltext

PROVIDERS' AUXILIARY STAFF ROLES IN TELEMEDICINE

Introduction

Each state has a different list of which providers may provide and bill for telemedical services. The common constants are medical doctors (MDs) and doctorsof osteopathy (DOs) as well as nurse practitioners (NPs), and physician assistants (PAs). Other states allow for paid services of therapists, psychologists, dieticians, and physical therapists.

Telenursing services, home health services, education, and patient follow-ups are usually not billable by themselves. Certain states, especially during COVID-19, allowed for the billing of these services. Please refer to your state's and federal web pages for the most up-to-date billing data for these services.

A lot of the amended rules and regulations end with the phrase "that this will end at the end of the Public Health Emergency (PHE)." This is very vague terminology and leads to a level of uncertainty as to what rules will change or end and when that may occur.

Providers

They must remember their duty to act and the ability to maintain standard of care. The provider is the first line of information technology (IT) support for themselves and patients. While they are not expected to be the IT expert, they should be able to navigate their computers, internet connections, and problem-solve for simple concerns.

What Providers Should Know

- Their state's regulations
- Which billing codes are acceptable
- How to approach billing coding concerns
- Navigate the chosen platform
- When and what prescriptions are appropriate to be ordered during an initial versus an established patient telemedical evaluation
- When and which codes their state allows them to bill for and patients should be scheduled for them appropriately
- How to self-advertise their telemedical and digital health services (American Medical Association, 2020, p. 115)

Overall, the clinician needs to become the jack-of-all-trades for telemedicine, especially if they are working remotely. There will likely not be the appropriate support person sitting right next to them, and they should not waste time trying to contact someone. Having a working knowledge of rules, regulations, IT, and billing guidelines will make their jobs easier and the patient flow smoother. Patients will also feel more comfortable with a clinician confident in their telemedical abilities.

NPs and PAs

While physician (MD and DO) rules and regulations are usually standard across state lines, NP and PA rules and regulations can vary. Many states follow the Nurse Practice Act and/or the laws regarding PAs, which are the key to how NPs and PAs can provide telemedical care in that state. However, some states stipulate how NPs and PAs can provide different care and bill for these services.

PA Roles

PA virtual care information usually follows a physician's recommendations and guidance. There is some information specific to PA telemedical care. However, the majority of these rules and regulations get lumped into those of the physician supervisors. COVID-specific laws tend to focus more on PA than NP regulations.

NP Roles

Most states do not have specific legislation regarding telemedical care to all providers, specifically NPs. To advance telemedical services, NPs in individual states should petition their state legislature to add these acts.

NP virtual care policies were put forth in an article in *Telehealth and Medicine Today* (Garber & Chike-Harris, 2019) in a table stating whether states have information in their various practice acts with specific regard to how it applies to NPs. Note that this is a guideline, and the full text of states' practice acts should be consulted to confirm the information.

Nurse Practice Act

The Nurse Practice Act is the state's governing document. It is published by the state's Board of Nursing and includes the scope of practice and any limitations or restrictions on the licensure of a registered nurse (RN) or advanced practice registered nurse (APRN). Very few states mention telehealth in the Nurse Practice Act.

Medical Practice Act

The Medical Practice Act is the state's governing document. It is published by the state's Board of Medical Examiners and includes the scope of practice and any limitations or restrictions on the licensure of MDs. Some states include DOs in this as well; others have their own Board of Osteopathic Physicians.

Some states also include PAs in this as well. Very few states mention information about telemedicine/telehealth.

Telehealth Act

Many states do not have an official Telehealth Act. For states that do have a Telehealth Act, this act would include what can or cannot be completed via telehealth. Prescriptions, providers, and other limitations and/or restrictions are usually mentioned in it.

Telehealth Position Statement

The telehealth position statement is a document that describes what telehealth and other electronic services are offered and how the state feels about telehealth helping fill the void and offering other services from an electronic point of view. This is usually in an effort to increase support and payment parity for telemedical and telehealth services.

TABLE 6.1 STATE TELEHEALTH REGULATION LOCATION

State	Nurse Practice Act	Medical Practice Act	Telehealth Act	APRN/ Nursing Advisory Options	Telehealth Position Statements
Alabama	N	N	N	N	Y
Alaska	N	N	Has some information, not directly involved with NP	Y	N

(continued)

TABLE 6.1 **STATE TELEHEALTH REGULATION LOCATION** (*CONTINUED*)

State	Nurse Practice Act	Medical Practice Act	Telehealth Act	APRN/ Nursing Advisory Options	Telehealth Position Statements
Arizona	N	N	Has some informa-tion, not directly involved with NP	N	N
Arkansas	N	N	Y	N	Y
California	N	N	Y	Y	N
Colorado	Y	N	Y	N	N
Connecti-cut	N	N	Y	N	N
Delaware	Y	N	N	N	N
Florida	N	N	N	N	Y
Georgia	N	N	Y	N	N
Hawaii	Y	N	Y	N	N
Idaho	N	N	Y	N	N

(*continued*)

TABLE 6.1 **STATE TELEHEALTH REGULATION LOCATION**
(*CONTINUED*)

State	Nurse Practice Act	Medical Practice Act	Telehealth Act	APRN/ Nursing Advisory Options	Telehealth Position Statements
Illinois	N	N	Y	N	N
Indiana	N	N	Y	N	N
Iowa	N	N	N	N	Y
Kansas	N	N	Y	N	N
Kentucky	Y	N	Y	N	N
Louisiana	N	N	Has some information, not directly involved with NP	N	N
Maine	N	N	Has some information, not directly involved with NP	N	N
Maryland	N	N	Y	N	N

(continued)

TABLE 6.1 **STATE TELEHEALTH REGULATION LOCATION**
(*CONTINUED*)

State	Nurse Practice Act	Medical Practice Act	Telehealth Act	APRN/ Nursing Advisory Options	Telehealth Position Statements
Massachu- setts	N	N	N	N	Has some informa- tion, not directly involved with NP
Michigan	Y	N	Y	N	N
Minnesota	Y	N	Y	N	N
Mississippi	N	N	N	N	Has some informa- tion, not directly involved with NP
Missouri	Y	N	Y	N	N
Montana	N	Has some informa- tion, not directly involved with NP	N	N	N
Nebraska	N	Y	Y	N	N

(*continued*)

TABLE 6.1 **STATE TELEHEALTH REGULATION LOCATION** (*CONTINUED*)

State	Nurse Practice Act	Medical Practice Act	Telehealth Act	APRN/ Nursing Advisory Options	Telehealth Position Statements
Nevada	N	N	Y	N	N
New Hamp-shire	Y	N	Y	Y	Y
New Jersey	N	N	Y	N	N
New Mexico	N	N	Y	N	N
New York	N	N	Y	Y	Y
North Carolina	N	N	Has some informa-tion, not directly involved with NP	Y	Y
North Dakota	N	N	Has some informa-tion, not directly involved with NP	N	N
Ohio	N	N	Y	Y	Y

(continued)

TABLE 6.1 **STATE TELEHEALTH REGULATION LOCATION** (*CONTINUED*)

State	Nurse Practice Act	Medical Practice Act	Telehealth Act	APRN/ Nursing Advisory Options	Telehealth Position Statements
Oklahoma	N	N	Has some information, not directly involved with NP	N	Y
Oregon	N	N	Has some information, not directly involved with NP	N	N
Pennsylvania	N	N	Y	Y	N
Rhode Island	N	N	Y	N	N
South Carolina	Y	N	Y	N	N
South Dakota	N	N	Has some information, not directly involved with NP	N	N
Tennessee	N	N	Y	N	N

(continued)

TABLE 6.1 **STATE TELEHEALTH REGULATION LOCATION** (*CONTINUED*)

State	Nurse Practice Act	Medical Practice Act	Telehealth Act	APRN/ Nursing Advisory Options	Telehealth Position Statements
Texas	N	N	Y	N	N
Utah	N	N	Y	Y	Y
Vermont	Y	N	Y	N	N
Virginia	N	N	Y	N	N
Washington	N	N	Y	N	N
West Virginia	N	N	Y	N	Y
Wisconsin	N	N	Y	N	N
Wyoming	N	N	Y	Y	N

APRN, advanced practice registered nurse; NP, nurse practitioner.

Physician Roles

Physician care and billing guidelines are usually standard. Advanced practice clinicians (APCs) performing these services should take the time at the beginning of their telemedicine practice to familiarize themselves with any modifications they need to make from in-person care to telemedical. The information and tables in this book should function as a guide, but the final answer comes from the Centers for Medicare and Medicaid Services, commercial payors, and state and federal legislation.

■ Auxiliary Staff Roles

Medical assistants, receptionists, and technology support staff have a vital role in the digital health world. Everything needs to be working at a high level for the successful implementation and execution of a telemedical solution. They should be knowledgeable in all aspects of digital healthcare as they function also in a role of a cheerleader for the platform and the digital health service of an organization.

An important role of all support staff is to explain and make sure the patients understand what digital health, telemedicine, and remote patient monitor are and what they entail. They should be well versed in its benefits and be conversant with patients, families, and potential patients about how much time and money it will save as well as the benefits of digital health to their own health.

The auxiliary support staff is the backbone of an organization. If they do not perform well in their roles and complete their responsibilities as they are directed, the whole system will falter. While this is true for in-person services, it takes on a whole new level for the digital platform. These staff members should be fully trained at the beginning of the service, and reeducation should be provided periodically throughout.

Training

The auxiliary staff should be properly trained in the electronic medical record (EMR) the telemedical platform, and the provider they work with. This allows for the continuation of the provider/patient relationship. Staff must be as familiar with the product as the provider is and, in some ways, even more so. They are the first line of IT support and the best problem-solvers for patients. They must be able to trouble-shoot and be able to communicate clearly to patients how to make the platform work quickly and efficiently.

Front Desk

The front desk staff change only slightly during this transition to the digital world.

Front desk responsibilities include the following:

- Verifying all patient information
  - In the case of new patients, inputting the information
- Contacting insurance companies to verify benefits (especially telemedical benefits)
- Scheduling follow-up appointments and assuring specialist consults are created

Medical Assistants (MAs)

The MA will still be responsible for collecting the appropriate medical data such as any vital signs the patient can collect at home (blood pressure, heart rate, glucose, pulse oximetry, temperature), updating the medical and surgical history, and recording any allergies and medications the patient is on.

Nurses

During a telehealth assessment, the nurse should complete their duties in the same way as they would in person. The platform also offers a perfect place to discuss how to handle emergency situations and allows for the intervention of care measures that would otherwise wait until the next office visit.

Nurse responsibilities include the following:

- Providing education about
  - Disease state
  - Overall health

- ☐ Medication
- ☐ Managing remote patient monitoring (RPM) devices
- ☐ How to appropriately schedule follow-up evaluations.
- ▨ If the patient is provided RPM supplies
  - ☐ Making sure that the patient is utilizing the products correctly, uploading the data to the provider correctly, and knows how to interpret their own data to stay as safe and healthy as possible

Office Manager and Administrator

The office manager and administrator carry the same responsibilities as in the office. For digital health, they are responsible for supporting medical assistants, schedulers, and providers. This position also becomes the problem-solver and the coordinator of all care measures. This will likely not differ from their in-person role and responsibilities.

Overall, the various roles of the digital health platform are important to its success. If each member of the team does not know their job or does not perform it to the top of their abilities, the success of the entire team will be in jeopardy.

It is also important to know the surrounding jobs as callouts and role changes can occur. This allows for cross-coverage and increases the overall success.

▨ References

American Medical Association. (2020). *AMA telehealth playbook.* www.ama-assn.org/system/files/2020-04/ama-telehealth-playbook.pdf

Garber, K. M., & Chike-Harris, K. E. (2019, June 28). Nurse practitioners and virtual care: A 50-state review of APRN telehealth law and policy. *Telehealth and Medicine Today, 4.* https://doi.org/10.30953/tmt.v4.136

LEGAL AND BILLING ISSUES

7

FEDERAL AND STATE LAWS RELATING TO TELEMEDICINE

Introduction

Legislation guiding and enforcing telemedicine and digital health as a whole is a dynamic feature of this aspect of medicine. While each state controls its own laws and guidelines, the federal government, and its various legislative bodies offer other legal twists and turns. The Centers for Medicare and Medicaid Services (CMS) provide the most data about what services they will or will not cover and what codes are required. State Medicaid and private insurers can be more cryptic. Some states also offer more concrete rules and regulations while others are a bit vaguer. Advanced practice clinicians (APCs), including nurse practitioners (NPs) and physician assistants (PAs), occasionally have different rules and regulations regarding billing and their ability to provide care. There is a table for this in the provider section.

Legislation for PAs tends to follow the physician regulations while NPs have vaguer information. In Michigan, PAs are billed under the supervising position, and in Pennsylvania, there are conflicting guidelines. In all states, however, medical doctors (MDs), doctors of osteopathy, NPs, and PAs can provide digital health services as listed in the table presented later. These tables should be used guidelines as individual state websites provide more detailed guides for coverage and billing requirements.

The laws regarding the establishment of a physician/provider relationship vary greatly. However, for all states, standards of care must be met, providers must act within their scope of practice, proper identification must be provided by the patient, the provider must be established, and the proper documentation of all relevant information must be completed (American Medical Association [AMA], 2020).

This is just a small example of the laws, regulations, and limitations for providers of digital health services. Each state has much more in-depth information about what services will be covered and paid for.

Possible limitations include:

- Location of the provider and patient (from office, home, nursing homes, and acute care hospital)
- Other services such as dietary and nursing visits
  - Might vary in coverage, legal liability, and payment structures
- Prescribing based upon telemedical visits (controlled and noncontrolled medications).

Which code or modifier must associate the current procedural terminology (CPT) code also varies. Some states do not cover telephonic codes or other CPT codes as defined by the CMS. A great resource for this is the Center for Connected Health Policy's State Telehealth Laws and Reimbursement Policies.

Alabama

- Patients must establish care in person.
- Patients must have seen someone in person first, but the patient can be seen digitally if they were referred from a face-to-face provider.
- Yearly face-to-face visits are required.

■ The provider must establish that the person is who they claim to be and that the diagnosis came via appropriate medical practices (history, exam, and diagnostic studies).

Modes of digital health allowed:

■ Live video (LV)

■ Remote patient monitoring(RPM)

NO parity laws
Specific telehealth consents required
Relevant State Guidelines and Laws

■ AAC 540-X-15-.09

■ AAC 540-X-15-.10

■ AAC 540-X-15-.11

Alaska

■ The medical board should have regulations that a provider who makes a diagnosis, treats, or prescribes must be initiated in person.

■ The medical board cannot impose disciplinary actions for treatments without a physical exam if they are located in the same state or the physician requests medical records.

■ Providers may not render a diagnosis solely based upon patient-supplied data.

Modes of digital health allowed:

■ LV

■ Store and forward (S/F)

■ RPM

NO parity laws
Specific telehealth consents NOT required
Relevant State Guidelines and Laws

- AS08.64.01 (6)
- AS 08.64.364
- 12 AAC 40.967 (27)

Arizona

- Relationships can be established via telemedicine, and prescriptions can be issued via telemedicine.
- The AZ Board of Osteopathic Examiners' telemedicine policy does not address the formation of the physician/patient relationship.

Modes of digital health allowed:

- LV
- S/F
- RPM

NO parity laws
Specific telehealth consents required
Relevant State Guidelines and Laws

- ARS 32.1401 (27) (ss) and (ww), ARS 32-1854 (48)
- ARS 36-3602

Arkansas

- Relationships can be established via telemedicine. No prescription can be prescribed unless a previous relationship exists.
- Under specific circumstances, such as emergency situations, telemedical relationships are allowed to be formed. Telemedicine relationships can also be formed for situations in which the standard of care can be met electronically.

Modes of digital health allowed:

- LV

NO parity laws
Specific telehealth consents required
Relevant State Guidelines and Laws

- ACA 17-80-403
- ACA 17-80-117
- ACA 17-80-404
- ACA 17-80-405
- ACA 17-80-406
- ACA 17-80-407
- ACA 17-80-401

California

- Relationships can be developed via telemedicine.
- Providers cannot prescribe Controlled Dangerous Substances (CDS) without a previously established relationship.

Modes of digital health allowed:

- LV
- S/F

Parity laws
Specific telehealth consents required
Relevant State Guidelines and Laws

- Cal. Bus. & Prof. Code 2290.5
- Cal. Bus. & Prof. Code 2242.1(a)
- Cal. Bus. & Prof. Code 4139-4135

Colorado

- The patient/provider relationship can be established via telemedicine as long as it conforms to the standards of practice.

Modes of digital health allowed:

- LV
- RPM

NO parity laws
Specific telehealth consents required
Relevant State Guidelines and Laws

- Colorado Medical Board (CMB) policy 40-3
- CMB policy 40-27

Connecticut

- A relationship between physician and patient can be established during real-time audio/visual communications with the provider's access to the patient's health information.
- No CDS can be prescribed unless certain circumstances are met—substance abuse therapy and so forth.

Modes of digital health allowed:

- LV
- S/F

NO parity laws
Specific telehealth consents required
Relevant State Guidelines and Laws

- Public Act 15-88 (2015)

Delaware

- The physician/patient relationship can be formed via telemedicine if the standard of care can be met.

Modes of digital health allowed:

- LV

Parity laws
Specific telehealth consents required
Relevant State Guidelines and Laws

- 24 Del. Code 1769D
- DE code, title 16 S4744

District of Columbia

- Physician/patient relationships can be established via real-time audio/video means with a full evaluation of all patient health records.

Modes of digital health allowed:

- LV

NO parity laws
Specific telehealth consents required
Relevant State Guidelines and Laws

- DC Medical Board Policy No 15-01
- DC Law 20-26; DC Official Code 31-3861

Florida

- Physicians and PAs can be established via telemedicine if the standard of care can be met and the patient's chart reflects decision-making, history, and physical.

Modes of digital health allowed:

- LV

NO parity laws
Specific telehealth consents NOT required
Relevant State Guidelines and Laws

- Florida Admin Code 64B8-9.0141
- Florida Admin Code 64B15-14.0081 (osteopaths)
- Florida Admin Code 64B15-14.0081

Georgia

- Physician, PA, and NP relationships with patients can be established electronically.
- However, they should attempt to have the patient seen face-to-face annually.

Modes of digital health allowed:

- LV
- S/F

Parity laws
Specific telehealth consents required
Relevant State Guidelines and Laws

- Code of Georgia Ann 360-3-.07

Hawaii

- Physician/patient relationships can be established via telemedicine with proper documentation and standard of care.

Modes of digital health allowed:

- LV

Parity laws
Specific telehealth consents NOT required
Relevant State Guidelines and Laws

- Haw. Rev. Stat 453-1.3
- Haw. Rev. Stat 329-1
- Haw. Rev. Stat 269-1
- Haw. Rev. Stat 346-1
- Haw. Rev. Stat 453-1.3

Idaho

- Physician/patient relationships can be established via telemedicine, and medications can be prescribed.

- CDS can only be prescribed in compliance.

Modes of digital health allowed:

- LV

NO parity laws
Specific telehealth consents required
Relevant State Guidelines and Laws

- Idaho Code Ann. 54-5606
- Idaho Code Ann. 54-1733
- Idaho Code Ann. 54-5607
- 21 U.S.C section 802(54)(A)

Illinois

- Physician/provider relationships are not addressed. It defers to medical judgment

Modes of digital health allowed:

- LV
- RPM

NO parity laws
Specific telehealth consents NOT required
Relevant State Guidelines and Laws

- 215 Ill. Comp Stat. Ann 5/356z.22(a)
- 225 Ill. Comp Stat Ann 60/49.5

Indiana

- Physician/patient relationships can be established electronically as long as the same standard of care as in-person care is met.
- CDS can only be prescribed if a previous visit was completed in person.

Modes of digital health allowed:

- LV
- RPM

NO parity laws
Specific telehealth consents NOT required
Relevant State Guidelines and Laws

- Indiana Code 25-1-9.5(7)
- Indiana Code 25-1-9.5(9)
- 844 IAC 5-8-1
- Indiana Code 25-1-9.5(8)
- Indiana Code 25-1-9.5(1)–(6)

Iowa

- Physician/patient relationships may be established electronically as long as the standard of care is met.
- Prescriptions can be issued after audio/video evaluation.

Modes of digital health allowed:

- LV

NO parity laws
Specific telehealth consents NOT required
Relevant State Guidelines and Laws

- Iowa Medical Board Rule 653-13.11 (147.148.272C)

Kansas

- Telemedicine can be utilized to establish a patient/provider relationship via a real-time audio/visual evaluation.

Modes of digital health allowed:

- LV
- RPM

NO parity laws
Specific telehealth consents required
Relevant State Guidelines and Laws

- KSA 2017 Supp. 40-2

Kentucky

- Physician/patient relationships can be established via telemedicine evaluation.

Modes of digital health allowed:

- LV

NO parity laws
Specific telehealth consents required
Relevant State Guidelines and Laws

- Kentucky Rev Stat Ann 311.597
- 907 KAR 3:170

Louisiana

- Physician/patient relationships can be established via telemedicine if the standard of care is met.
- CDS can be prescribed without an in-person evaluation.

Modes of digital health allowed:

- LV
- RPM

Specific telehealth consents required
NO parity laws
Relevant State Guidelines and Laws

- Louisiana Rev. Stat. 37:1276.1
- LRS 37:1271

Maine

- Physician/patient relationships can be established via real-time telemedicine.

Modes of digital health allowed:

- LV
- RPM

NO parity laws
Specific telehealth consents required
Relevant State Guidelines and Laws

- 22 MRSA 3173-H
- 24-A Maine Rev. Stat. Ann. 4316

Maryland

- Physician/patient relationships can be established via a real-time telemedical evaluation.

Modes of digital health allowed:

- LV
- S/F
- RPM

NO parity laws
Specific telehealth consents required
Relevant State Guidelines and Laws

- Code of Maryland Regulations (COMAR) 10.32.05.05
- COMAR 10.32.05.01

Massachusetts

- Physician/patient relationships can be established via a real-time telemedical evaluation.

Modes of digital health allowed:

- LV

NO parity laws
Specific telehealth consents NOT required
Relevant State Guidelines and Laws

- Board of Registration of Medicine Policy 03-06
- 243 CMR 2.01

Michigan

- Providers must have a previously established relationship with patients.
- In-person follow-up care should be available.

Modes of digital health allowed:

- LV

NO parity laws
Specific telehealth consents required
Relevant State Guidelines and Laws

- MI compiled Laws 333.17751; 16285
- Senate Bill No. 270 Statue 7303a
- Michigan Insurance Code 500.3476

Minnesota

- A physician/patient relationship can be established via telemedicine.
- A full evaluation must be completed prior to prescribing.

Modes of digital health allowed:

- LV
- S/F
- RPM

Parity laws
Specific telehealth consents required
Relevant State Guidelines and Laws

- Minnesota Stat. Ann. 147.033
- Minn. Stat. Ann 151.37 Minn. Stat. Ann. 147.033 (1)(1)

Mississippi

- Physician/patient relationships can be established via telemedicine.
- CDS can be prescribed after the completion of a visit.
- Standard of care must be met.

Modes of digital health allowed:

- LV
- RPM

NO parity laws
Specific telehealth consents required
Relevant State Guidelines and Laws

- MS Code Ann. 41-29-137
- MS Code 83-9-351

Missouri

- Physician/patient relationships can be established via telemedicine if standards of care are met.

Modes of digital health allowed:

- LV
- RPM

NO parity laws
Specific telehealth consents required
Relevant State Guidelines and Laws

- RSMo 191.1146
- RSMo 191.1145

Montana

- Physician/patient relationships are not addressed in the state code.

Modes of digital health allowed:

- LV

NO parity laws
Specific telehealth consents NOT required
Relevant State Guidelines and Laws
- Montana code Ann. 37-3-102(13)

Nebraska

- A physician or PA may establish a patient/provider relationship via telemedicine and can prescribe using telemedicine.

Modes of digital health allowed:

- LV
- RPM

NO parity laws
Specific telehealth consents required

Relevant State Guidelines and Laws

- Rev. Stat. Nebraska Ann. 38-2001
- Rev. Stat. Nebraska Ann. 71-8501
- Rev. Stat. Nebraska Ann. 38-2001(6)
- Rev. Stat. Nebraska Ann. 38-105

Nevada

- Physician/patient relationships may be established via telemedicine.
- Standard of care must be met.

Modes of digital health allowed:

- LV
- S/F

NO parity laws
Specific telehealth consents NOT required
Relevant State Guidelines and Laws

- Nevada Rev. Stat. 633-165
- Nevada Rev. Stat. 630.020
- Nevada Rev. Stat. An. 633.171 (osteopath)
- NV Bill AB 292

New Hampshire

- Physician/patient relationships may be established via real-time audio/visual telemedicine.
- A CDS cannot be prescribed if it is an opioid.
- Non-opioids can be prescribed by certain providers with whom an in-person relationship exists.

Modes of digital health allowed:

- LV

NO parity laws
Specific telehealth consents required
Relevant State Guidelines and Laws

- RSA 329:1-c
- NH Bill SB 84
- RSA 22-1

New Jersey

- Physician/patient relationships may be established via telemedicine.
- Out-of-state consultation may occur using telemedicine.
- Standard of care must be met.
- Schedule 2 CDS cannot be prescribed via telemedicine until after an in-person evaluation occurs and is completed every 3 months.
- Stimulants for minors using audio/video real-time evaluation can be completed via telemedicine with parental/guardian consent.

Modes of digital health allowed:

- LV

Parity laws
Specific telehealth consents required
Relevant State Guidelines and Laws

- R.S. 45:9-18
- NJ Statue C.45:1-62
- NJ Statute C. 45:1-63

New Mexico

- A real-time telemedicine encounter can institute a relationship between provider and patient.
- Medical records must be generated.

Modes of digital health allowed:

- LV
- S/F

Parity laws
Specific telehealth consents required
Relevant State Guidelines and Laws

- New Mexico Admin Code 16:10.8.7
- New Mexico Admin Code 16:10.8.8
- N.M.S.A./1978, 24-25-3 (osteopath)

New York

- Telemedicine can be used to establish a patient/provider relationship.

Modes of digital health allowed:

- LV
- S/F
- RPM

NO parity laws
Specific telehealth consents required
Relevant State Guidelines and Laws

- NY Medical Board of Professional Medical Conduct
- NY public Health Law 2999-cc

North Carolina

- Physician/provider relationships can be created via telemedicine.
- Prescribing can only be completed when a relationship exists.

Modes of digital health allowed:

- LV

NO parity laws
Specific telehealth consents NOT required
Relevant State Guidelines and Laws

- North Colorado Medical Board (NCMB) Position Statement on Telemedicine
- NCMB Position Statement on Contact with Patients before Prescribing
- NCMB Position Statement on Telemedicine

North Dakota

- Patient/provider relationships can be established via telemedicine if the standard of care can be met.
- Prescribing can only be completed after a relationship exists.

Modes of digital health allowed:

- LV

NO parity laws
Specific telehealth consents NOT required
Relevant State Guidelines and Laws

- ND Admin Code 50-2-15
- ND Cent. Code 19-02.1-15-1

Ohio

- Physician/provider relationships can be established via telemedicine as long as the standard of care is met.
- Prescribing after a relationship is established is allowed.

Modes of digital health allowed:
- LV

NO parity laws
Specific telehealth consents required
Relevant State Guidelines and Laws

- State Medical Board of Ohio Position Statement on Telemedicine
- 4731-11-09

Oklahoma

- Physician/patient relationships may be established via telemedicine; this can include S/F.
- Standard of care must be met.
- Health Information Privacy and Portability Act (HIPAA) compliance must be maintained.

Modes of digital health allowed:

- LV

NO parity laws
Specific telehealth consents required
Relevant State Guidelines and Laws

- O.A.C. 478.1:59
- O.A.C. 435: 10-7-4
- O.A.C. 435: 10-7-13
- O.A.C. 478:59
- O.A.C. 435: 10-1-4

Oregon

- The physician can use judgment to establish care via telemedicine.

Modes of digital health allowed:

- LV
- RPM

NO parity laws
Specific telehealth consents required
Relevant State Guidelines and Laws

- Oregon Admin. Rules Comp. 847-025-0000
- Oregon Medical Board (OMB) Statement of Philosophy

Pennsylvania

- No specific statue
- PA does not address the formation of the patient/ provider relationship.

Modes of digital health allowed:

- LV

NO parity laws
Specific telehealth consents required
Relevant State Guidelines and Laws

Rhode Island

- Physician/patient relationships can be established via telemedicine.
- A sufficient platform should be in place, and the standard of care must be met.

Modes of digital health allowed:

- LV

NO parity laws
Specific telehealth consents required
Relevant State Guidelines and Laws

- Rhode Island Board of Medical Licensure and Discipline
- Guidelines for the Appropriate Use of Telemedicine

South Carolina

- Physician/patient relationships can be established via telemedicine if the standard of care should be met.

- HIPAAand Health Information Technology for Economic and Clinical Health Act information must be maintained.

Modes of digital health allowed:

- LV

- RPM

NO parity laws
Specific telehealth consents required
Relevant State Guidelines and Laws

- South Carolina Admin. Code 40-47-37

- South Carolina Admin. Code 40-47-113

- SC Board of Medical Examiners

- SCAC 40-47-20(52)

South Dakota

- No specific guidelines regarding relationship

- Must be licensed in South Dakota

Modes of digital health allowed:

- LV

NO parity laws
Specific telehealth consents NOT required
Relevant State Guidelines and Laws

- SD Codified Laws 36-4-41

Tennessee

- Telemedicine can be used to establish a physician/provider relationship.

- S/F can be used.

- Appropriate medical records must be maintained.
- Mutual consent to the platform must occur.

Modes of digital health allowed:

- LV
- S/F

NO parity laws
Specific telehealth consents required
Relevant State Guidelines and Laws

- Rules of Tennessee Board of Medical Examiners 0880-02.16
- Ten Code. Ann. 63-1-155(b)
- Ten Code. Ann. 63-1-155 (osteopath)
- Ten Code. Ann. 63-1-155(a)(2) and 63-1-155
- Tenn Code 56-7-1002(6)
- Rules of Tenn Board of Medical Examiners 0880-02(1)

Texas

- Telemedicine can be used to establish a relationship between physician and patient.

Modes of digital health allowed:

- LV
- S/F
- RPM

NO parity laws
Specific telehealth consents required
Relevant State Guidelines and Laws

- Texas Admin Code 174.6
- Occupations Code 11.004, 006 and 008
- Occupations Code 562.056

- TAC 174.2
- Occupations Code 111.001

Utah

- Telemedicine can be used to establish a patient/ provider relationship.
- Standard of care must be met.

Modes of digital health allowed:

- LV
- RPM

NO parity laws
Specific telehealth consents required
Relevant State Guidelines and Laws

- Utah Code Ann. 26-60-101

Vermont

- Physician/provider relationships can be formed via telemedicine if the standard of care is met.

Modes of digital health allowed:

- LV
- RPM

NO parity laws
Specific telehealth consents required
Relevant State Guidelines and Laws

- Vermont Board of Medical Practice Policy of Telemedicine

Virginia

- Patient/provider relationships may be formed via telemedicine if both sides consent and the standard of care is met.

■ CDS can be prescribed once a relationship is established.

Modes of digital health allowed:

■ LV

■ S/F

■ RPM

NO parity laws
Specific telehealth consents required
Relevant State Guidelines and Laws

■ Guidance Document 85-12: Telemedicine

■ Code of Virginia 54.1-3303

■ VA Code 38.2-3418.16

Washington

■ Provider/patient relationships can be established via telemedicine unless circumstances require an in-person evaluation.

Modes of digital health allowed:

■ LV

■ S/F

■ RPM

NO parity laws
Specific telehealth consents required
Relevant State Guidelines and Laws

■ MD2014-03: Telemedicine Guidelines

■ RCW 48.43.735

West Virginia

■ Physician/patient relationships can be established via telemedicine as long as it is not through audio or text only. Must be real-time audio/visual.

- Standard of care must be met.
- Schedule 2 CDS cannot be prescribed.

Modes of digital health allowed:

- LV

NO parity laws
Specific telehealth consents required
Relevant State Guidelines and Laws

- WV Medical Practice Act 30-3-13a(c), 301412d(c)
- WV Medical Practice Act 30-3-13a(d), 301412d(d)
- WV Medical Practice Act 30-3-13a(e), 301412d(e)
- WV Medical Practice Act 30-3-13a(g), 301412d(g)
- WV Medical Practice Act 30-3-13a(h), 301412d(h)
- WV Medical Practice Act 30-3-13a(j), 301412d(j)
- WV Board of Medicine and Osteopath Medicine Position Statement

Wisconsin

- Patient/physician relationships can be established via telemedicine.
- Standard of practice must be met.

Modes of digital health allowed:

- LV

NO parity laws
Specific telehealth consents required
Relevant State Guidelines and Laws

- Chapter Med 24

Wyoming

- Patient/physician relationships can be established via telemedicine.

- Professional standards must be met.

Modes of digital health allowed:

- LV

NO parity laws
Specific telehealth consents required
Relevant State Guidelines and Laws

- 33-13-03 Powers of licensure boards
- WY BOM Rules and Reg Ch 1(3)(yy)
- WY stat. Ann. 33-26-102

Note: All information was collected from the individual state practice websites.

What Providers Need to Know

Providers, administrators, and staff should be familiar with the laws concerning digital health:

- What services are covered
- How to properly code and bill
- What modifiers to utilize
- What can be completed via an initial patient evaluation versus the need for being an established patient
- Prescribing rules and regulations

All providers and staff should be properly licensed, obtain appropriate consent for procedures, and provide appropriate security measures. To protect providers and staff, the organization should look into appropriate malpractice coverage. Patients are protected by securing HIPAA protocols.

States and the CMS recommend proper cybersecurity guidelines for the protection of HIPAA information over a digital platform. Ultimately, it is the priority of providers and staff to assure that patients understand how to protect themselves and their information. For example, if a patient is completing their telemedical evaluation in public, the provider should suggest that the encounter be completed at another time.

Cybersecurity protocol recommendations:

- Appropriate-level security protocols
- Only specific portals open on a server
- Appropriate biometric access devices
- Changing of security codes on a regular basis

Consent forms may need to be adjusted to cover telemedical, telehealth, and RPM services. As with any other informed consent forms, the patient must be aware of any risks and benefits of the platform and the evaluation that would be completed.

Examples of specific information in the consent form include:

- Cyberattack risks
- HIPAA protection protocols
- Proper environments for the evaluation to be completed
- What is appropriate for telemedical services

The AMA released an opinion paper (2020) about which documents should be completed and maintained by the practice when implementing a digital health platform.

TABLE 7.1 **DOCUMENTS FOR STARTING A DIGITAL HEALTH DEPARTMENT OR PRACTICE**

Legal Documents	Definition
Business Associate Agreement	A document that states all parties associated with the business will interact with HIPAA materials will be compliant with standing protocols. This also outlines the penalties for breaking these protocols
Master Service Agreement	A document outlining the business relationship
Scope of work/price quote	A document that states the specific work with its timing, cost, timelines, and what will be delivered
Purchase order	A document stating the price for services and products
Financial audit reports	A document about the financial health of the organization
Confidentiality agreement/NDA	This states the information the can and cannot be shared with the vendor/organization but not anyone else
W-9 form	A document regarding the taxes of the vendor and their tax ID number

HIPAA, Health Insurance Portability and Accountability Act; NDA, nondisclosure agreement.
Source: American Medical Association. (2020). *AMA telehealth playbook*. www.ama-assn.org/system/files/2020-04/ama-telehealth-play book.pdf

The AMA lists documents proving that the products are safe, approved for use, and proper insurance coverage and licenses are available.

TABLE 7.2 **ADDITIONAL DOCUMENTS FOR STARTING A DIGITAL HEALTH DEPARTMENT OR PRACTICE**

Validation Documents	Definition
IT security and risk assessment	A document of the vendor's security procedures
510(k) clearance	Proof that the FDA has determined the medical device to be safe and effective
Liability insurance	Proper insurance to cover malpractice, bodily injury, property damage, lawsuit, and medical expenses
Medical licenses for providers and applicable staff	Appropriate licenses from the state or other governing body to practice medicine, nursing, and so forth in the state they serve
Third-party audit	A document to prove validation of compliance with HIPAA and other security protocols

FDA, Food and Drug Administration; HIPAA, Health Information Privacy and Portability Act; IT, information technology.
Source: American Medical Association. (2020). *AMA telehealth playbook.* www.ama-assn.org/system/files/2020-04/ama-telehealth-play book.pdf

◼ Reference

American Medical Association. (2020). *AMA telehealth playbook.* www.ama-assn.org/system/files/2020-04/ama-telehealth-play book.pdf

8

BILLING AND REIMBURSEMENT FOR TELEMEDICINE

◼ Introduction

While we are all in this field to help the patients under our care, billing is a necessary evil. Without the constant inflow of revenue from payors, governments, and patients (copays, deductibles) we could not offer the services we do. Medicare and Medicaid plans usually reimburse for digital health services differently than commercial payors. Some commercial insurances do not cover digital health services at all, while others offer incentives for these care modalities (reduced copay or no copay, reduced deductible).

◼ Parity Laws

Parity laws are acts of legislation that force payors to pay for telemedical services as they would for an in-person exam. There is an up-to-date table of states that have passed this legislation in the state and federal laws chapter. As stated, there are parity laws in almost all states. During the COVID-19 pandemic, further legislation was enacted. States that do not already have permanent legislation will still need to determine what laws and rules will remain once the public health emergency is lifted. While some states have enacted this legislation, insurance companies can still choose to pay the rate they determine appropriate. It should be stressed to the patient that this may not affect copays and deductibles as each insurance plan and policy may differ.

▨ The Digital Medicine Payment Advisory Group

The Digital Medicine Payment Advisory Group is a subsidiary of the American Medical Association (AMA) that assists with coding and helps to improve reimbursements. This is completed by

- ▨ creating and releasing information about clinical telemedical technology,
- ▨ reviewing billing and procedural codes to determine their usefulness in digital medicine and the application to proper patient care,
- ▨ providing education to payors and executives for appropriate coverage of digital healthcare services, and
- ▨ continuing the appropriate use and application of digital medicine.

(AMA, 2020)

Ultimately this group assists in making the digital experience happy and productive for patients, consumers, business specialists and clinicians.

▨ Guidelines for Billing

Guidelines for billing telemedical evaluations are similar to in-person evaluations. The two main differences are billing based upon time spent and documenting it as a telemedical evaluation: the platform used and the type of visit. The type of visit would be audio only (telephonic codes), audio/visual either store and forward (asynchronous) or real time (synchronous).

Overall, the same code that would be used to bill for an in-person evaluation is the code used for a telemedical encounter. To denote the usage of digital services, use the modifier "GT" for government payors (Medicare and Medicaid) or the modifier "95" for commercial payors. While in-person evaluation and coding usually rely on systems evaluated, telemedical assessments can be billed based upon time spent with patients. This can include, but not be limited to, counseling, education, and assessing and referring patients to appropriate specialists. Medical complexity can also be factored into the billing code and must be documented appropriately. To bill the code based upon time, the time spent in all aspects of care must also be clearly documented.

TABLE 8.1 **CPT BILLING CODES FOR CARE SERVICES**

New Patient		Established Patient	
CPT	Time	CPT	Time
99201	10 minutes	99211	5 minutes
99202	20 minutes	99212	10 minutes
99203	30 minutes	99213	15 minutes
99204	45 minutes	99214	25 minutes
99205	60 minutes	99215	40 minutes

CPT, Current Procedural Terminology.
Source: From American Medical Association. (2020). *AMA telehealth playbook.* https://www.ama-assn.org/system/files/2020-04/ama-telehealth-playbook.pdf.

▓ Medicare and Medicaid

After the Centers for Medicare and Medicaid Services (CMS) approved coverage of digital medicine billing around 2017, coding and reimbursement for digital health services vastly improved. Reimbursement for Medicare services can be tricky. The patient may have to be in a rural area and have difficulty obtaining medical services through other means. This was discontinued during the COVID-19 pandemic and at the time of writing has yet to be reverted to pre-COVID billing patterns. For commercial payors, the rules of patient location are more relaxed. This allows for greater coverage and ease of use for these services. Self-paying patients have no boundaries for services.

Wellness Visit Codes

Medicare offers annual wellness visit codes for telemedical exams. These must be completed in real-time audio/video synchronized evaluations. There are very few circumstances in which this code should be utilized. Providers should only perform a complete physical exam over telemedicine if there is no other choice or if the patient has access to specialized digital tools that allow for a full and proper physical exam.

TABLE 8.2 **MEDICARE WELLNESS CPT CODES**

Code	Description
G0438	Initial annual wellness visit
G0349	Subsequent visit

CPT, Current Procedural Terminology
Source: From American Medical Association. (2020). *AMA telehealth playbook.* https://www.ama-assn.org/system/files/2020-04/ama-telehealth-playbook.pdf.

Check-In Billing Codes

Medicare does have check-in billing codes. These can be utilized if the patient does not have an office visit within 7 days; otherwise, this visit is bundled into the office visit billing.

These codes are as follows:

TABLE 8.3 **MEDICARE CPT CHECK-IN CODES**

Code	Description
CPT 99421	Online digital evaluation and management for an established patient for up to 7 days (MD, DO, NP, PA)
	5–10 minutes
CPT 99422	11–20 minutes
CPT 99423	21 or more minutes
CPT 98970	Qualified nonphysician health care professional online digital assessment (physical/occupational therapy, speech pathologist, psychologist)
	5–10 minutes
CPT 98971	11–20 minutes
CPT 98972	21 or more minutes

(continued)

TABLE 8.3 **MEDICARE CPT CHECK-IN CODES (*CONTINUED*)**

Code	Description
HCPCS G2012	Brief communication technology–based service (can be completed by MD, DO, NP, PA). This cannot originate from a related service within the previous 7 days or the future 24 hours.
	5–10 minutes

CPT, Current Procedural Terminology; DO, doctor of osteopathy; MD medical doctor; NP, nurse practitioner; PA, physician assistant.
Note: CPT 98970-98972 were updated in 2020 to replace HCPCS code G2061-G2063.
Source: From American Medical Association. (2020). *AMA telehealth playbook.* https://www.ama-assn.org/system/files/2020-04/ama-telehealth-playbook.pdf.

For these services to be billable, the patient must have signed consent on file and be an established patient of the provider evaluating them. The patient and the provider must interact via real-time audio and video conversation. Audio-only calls (i.e., telephone conversations) are not allowed to be billed for these services. However, during the COVID-19 pandemic, the billing of audio-only visits was allowed.

Remote Patient Monitoring Codes

Remote patient monitoring codes became billable at the beginning of January 2018. These devices allow for patient-collected information to be sent electronically to their providers or other healthcare professionals.

These types of visits also require the patient to be an established patient of the practice and have advanced signed consent. The codes can only be billed every 30 days and can be combined with chronic care management codes (CPT 99487-99490).

TABLE 8.4 **REMOTE PATIENT MONITORING CODES**

Code	Description
CPT 99453	Initial setup and education of use for remote monitoring of physiologic parameters (weight, glucose, bp, temp, etc.)
CPT 99454	Device supply with daily recordings and transmissions. Can be billed every 30 days
CPT 99457	Remote monitoring and treatment plans for the healthcare provider. Billable monthly
	Patient and provider must communicate at least 20 minutes
CPT 99458	Each additional 20 minutes of interaction of patient and provider
CPT 99091	Collection and interpretation of data that has been evaluated and interpreted by a qualified medical provider. Minimum of 30 minutes every 30 days

CPT, Current Procedural Terminology
Source: From American Medical Association. (2020). *AMA telehealth playbook.* https://www.ama-assn.org/system/files/2020-04/ama-telehealth-playbook.pdf.

Telephone Evaluation and Management Codes

As previously stated, telephone evaluation and management of Medicare patients were deemed nonbillable as per CMS guidelines. During the COVID-19 pandemic, these rules were relaxed. At the time of writing, these rules had yet to be

TABLE 8.5 **TELEPHONE EVALUATION CPT CODES**

Code	Description
CPT 99487	Two or more conditions expected to last 12 months
	60 minutes of clinical staff time by a qualified provider
	Can be billed monthly
CPT 99489	Additional 30 minutes of time
CPT 99491	Chronic care services provided by a qualified healthcare practitioner, at least 30 minutes
	Must include a condition lasting over 12 months, significant risk of death/exacerbation

CPT, Current Procedural Terminology
Source: From American Medical Association. (2020). *AMA telehealth playbook.* https://www.ama-assn.org/system/files/2020-04/ama-telehealth-playbook.pdf.

reinstituted or revised. Private payors may cover telephonic evaluations of their patients.

These must be completed for an established patient, parent, or guardian. They cannot be billed within 7 days of a previous encounter with the provider using the same diagnostic or procedure codes. These codes can also not be billed if the telephone encounter leads to another type of evaluation within 24 hours.

TABLE 8.6 **CMS COLLABORATION CODES**

Code	Description
CPT 99441	Telephonic evaluation and management by a qualified medical provider (MD, DO, NP, PA)
	5–10 minutes
CPT 99442	11–20 minutes
CPT 99443	21–30 minutes

CMS, Centers for Medicare and Medicaid Services; DO, doctor of osteopathy; MD, medical doctor; NP, nurse practitioner; PA, physician assistant.
Source: From American Medical Association. (2020). *AMA telehealth playbook.* https://www.ama-assn.org/system/files/2020-04/ama-telehealth -playbook.pdf.

Interprofessional Collaboration Codes

Collaboration between medical professionals can also be billed under CMS guidelines. This allows for coordinated care across the specialties for the benefit of the patient. This especially benefits rural communities where the appropriate specialist, therapist, dietician, or other consultant is geographically remote.

In-Patient Care Codes

If a patient requires in-patient care at an acute care hospital or skilled nursing facility, Medicare has codes available for these types of electronic encounters as well.

The American Academy of Family Practice (AAFP) has a great flow chart of billing codes that conveys how, when,

TABLE 8.7 **IN-PATIENT BILLING CODES**

Code	Description
CPT 99446	Interprofessional audio or audio/visual collaboration and management of a specialist provider with a verbal and written report to the primary care provider
	5–10 minutes
CPT 99447	11–20 minutes
CPT 99448	21–30 minutes
CPT 99449	31 or more minutes
CPT 99452	Interprofessional electronic referral by the treating physician and specialist
	30 minutes

CPT, Current Procedural Terminology
Source: From American Medical Association. (2020). *AMA telehealth playbook.* https://www.ama-assn.org/system/files/2020-04/ama-telehealth -playbook.pdf.

and which codes to use. The AAFP also states that nine states require Medicaid only to pay for digital health services. Forty-one states will pay for both Medicaid and private insurance. Only fourteen states will pay for store-and-forward telemedical services, and only 22 will pay for remote patient monitoring services (AAFP, 2020).

TABLE 8.8 **ED AND IN-PATIENT BILLING CODES**

ED or Initial inpatient		Skilled Nursing Facility Follow-Up Visits	
G0425	Telehealth Consults ED or initial in-patient 30 minutes	G0406	Follow up inpatient either acute care hospital or SNF
			15 minutes
G0426	Telehealth Consults ED or initial in-patient 50 minutes	G0407	Follow up inpatient either acute care hospital or SNF
			25 minutes
G0427	Telehealth Consults ED or initial inpa-tient/SNF 70 minutes	G0408	Follow up inpatient either acute care hospital or SNF
			35 minutes

ED, emergency department; SNF, skilled nursing facility.
Source: From American Medical Association. (2020). *AMA telehealth playbook.* https://www.ama-assn.org/system/files/2020-04/ama-telehealth -playbook.pdf.

To determine if a televisit is a valid type of visit, first the team must determine if there is a need for the telemedical services to be in real time (synchronous) or saved and forwarded to the clinical team (asynchronous). From there, the clinician should determine if the visit is telemedical appropriate (i.e., not a complaint that requires a full physical exam or other situation in which the standard of care cannot be met electronically). Appropriate coding by the clinician should occur based upon the earlier charts and the time and complexity of the evaluation.

References

AAFP. (2020). *A virtual visit algorithm: how to differentiate and code telehealth visits, e-visits, and virtual check-ins.* https://www.aafp.org/journals/fpm/blogs/inpractice/entry/telehealth_algorithm.html

American Medical Association. (2020). *AMA telehealth implementation playbook.* https://www.ama-assn.org/system/files/2020-04/ama-telehealth-playbook.pdf

THE TELEMEDICINE VISIT

9

EVALUATING YOUR DIGITAL HEALTH APPROACH TO PATIENTS

Introduction

An evaluation of your digital health platform is key to the success of the program. Is the program profitable? Are patients and providers satisfied? These are just two of the questions that should be assessed periodically. The answers should be accepted without judgment and fear of punishment. The only way to grow and scale the program is to assess what is not working and adjust remove, or otherwise address concerns. Just as we evaluate our medical or business interventions, we must evaluate our digital health programs. This is usually completed at short-, medium- and long-term intervals.

Short-Term Goals: Usually measured in a period of 3 to 6 months

- Establish the focus for digital health at your practice (i.e., on-demand care, chronic care)
- Establish the management, support, and clinical team
- Decide upon the platform

Medium-Term Goals: Usually 6 to 12 months

- ■ Evaluation by clinical and administrative leaders for the success of the platform
- ■ Metrics can include fiscal, patient and provider satisfaction

Long-Term Goals: Usually 1 to 2 years

- ■ Metrics will be similar to the medium-term goals
- ■ Expansion and scaling of the platform

Different institutions will employ different methodologies to institute and initiate their short-, medium- and long-term goals. A common method is the Plan, Do, Study, Act methodology:

- ■ Plan what needs to be accomplished.
- ■ Do whatever it takes to complete the task.
- ■ Study the final product to determine if the intended outcome was met.
- ■ Act in accordance with what you find in the study phase.

There are other implementation and evaluation methods available, and this is just one that can allow for an organization to successfully implement a digital health solution.

Overall, this integration will be painful, but all growth comes with growing pains. Proper education, implementation and close follow-ups with the personnel performing day-to-day tasks should ensure a comfortable transition to the digital world. There needs to be close attention paid to each member inside of the organization.

The clinical and administrative leadership should work together to confirm that all aspects of the care team are doing their jobs and meeting their goals. There should be periodic checks to assure that nothing gets out of hand.

Metrics for Evaluation

Benefits to Patients

Benefits to the patient can be determined by their satisfaction with the platform the provider, return visits, and verbal recommendations to friends and family (see patient survey sample in Appendix D).

Medical Outcomes

Medical outcomes can be evaluated by the reduction in co-morbidities, the increased ability to perform activities of daily living, stricter compliance with dietary and medication management, and the reduction in complications of the patient's diagnosis.

Reimbursement and Reduction of Costly Services

A digital health program should also be evaluated based upon reimbursement and reduction in higher cost medical services like emergency department visits and admissions to inpatient and skilled nursing facilities. Costs can be further evaluated by reduced no-pay visits and canceled visits. The billing department should evaluate the revenue cycle monthly or quarterly and report to the executive team.

Provider Satisfaction

Provider satisfaction can be measured by decreased burnout, decreased appointment duration, and increased compliance to care plans.

Operations

Operations can be evaluated by how well the platform integrates into the organization's workflow.

◼ Frequently Encountered Areas for Improvement

Internally

When the problems or concerns come from within the leaders of the department in question, administrative or clinical, should find out if this is an education (or lack thereof) problem, software or hardware issue, or any other aspect that needs to be addressed. Reeducating the relevant staff, updating hardware, or adjusting workflow may all increase the quality and satisfaction of the program. Information technology (IT) may need to intervene and update hardware and internet connections to allow for the best quality digital interactions.

The Platform

When the problem comes from the platform, the organization should lean on the vendor providing the software. If needed, the organization can fall back on their contract to make proper updates, address hardware or software problems or offer solutions to make the platform more user-friendly. There should always be the means of contacting a representative of the vendor's IT team during all hours of the organization's care delivery periods. The vendor should make every effort to live up to its contract and the quality of service promised during the initial vetting stage. Most vendors should embrace the feedback of an organization as this allows for them to grow and be more marketable to other organizations.

Patient Education

If the problem is patient understanding, appropriate measures should be instituted to aid the patients in any areas of concern:

- ■ Is there a need for a patient ambassador or other role to aid in educating the patient?
- ■ Could other electronic means of appointment reminders like confirmation texts, emails, and/or phone calls minimize late visits or no-shows?

The patient may also need a pre-visit instruction of what is the appropriate technology to complete this evaluation (device with camera, appropriate internet speed). Time, effort, and frustration could also be alleviated by confirming the proper software has been downloaded prior to their appointment time (AMA, 2020, p. 89).

■ Continuous Quality Improvement

Once an evaluation of each side of the platform (vendor, patient, staff, organization, provider) is completed, time should be taken to listen and hear what everyone has to say to properly update and make adjustments to perfect the digital services. Improvements will always be required, workflow adjusted, software updated, and personnel reeducated. This is a part of life and how we grow as an organization. If a digital health platform is to be successful, errors must be worked out and the team learns how to make the flow smoother and more efficient. This will not be an easy process to start, but it is a necessary one. Were the deleted changes fully deleted or just moved?

■ Reference

American Medical Association. (2020). *AMA telehealth implementation playbook.* https://www.ama-assn.org/system/files/2020-04/ama-telehealth-playbook.pdf

TELEMEDICINE AND REMOTE VISIT ETIQUETTE WITH PATIENTS

Introduction

Proper visit etiquette makes a potentially uncomfortable situation more comfortable. As always with a provider–patient relationship, the comfort of both parties is key. The interaction via a digital platform should be conducted as if the provider werein the room with the patient. We are still professionals even if we are sitting in the comfort of our own home. The patient's sense of "Is this person caring about me or am I a number to them?" can be affected by the smallest characteristic of the evaluation and interaction.

Many patients, especially the elderly, may have no previous interaction via digital means. This does start the exchange at a disadvantage, but with kindness, compassion, and understanding, as well as the appropriate dress and mannerisms, the patient may be swayed to enjoy and embrace this medium for healthcare delivery.

The Environment and Camera Focus

Call center or receptionist staff should educate patients about the proper environment in the pre-visit period. The patient has the responsibility of providing an appropriate environment for themselves, free of distractions and with minimal outside noise. Occasionally, people present for their telemedical evaluation in public or at work. This is unacceptable as it is not Health Information Privacy and Portability Act compliant and does not offer the ability for them to focus on the provider. They should also be gently instructed to keep interruptions to a minimum.

For the provider, the camera should frame their face and upper body and limit the extraneous noise and background sounds. Remember, the patient will likely be able to see the room behind the provider. The provider should not have anything offensive in their home, office, or wherever they are providing care. However, there is the possibility that something that one considers art and appropriate may not be the same for someone else (nude or expressive art, etc.). Distractions on either side of the evaluation, for example, children, pets and co-workers, should be minimalized. This may not be 100% possible, but precautions should be in place to ensure a calm, quiet environment.

▉ Body Language

Body language is another important component of the encounter. The provider must appear to be engaged in the interaction. The same way we would comport ourselves in an in-person exam should be the same as a digital health assessment. Wandering eyes convey a message of boredom or a lack of interest, and being slumped over in the chair, having one's crossed arms or other uninterested gestures decrease the quality of the digital health exam.

Our patients are coming to us for comfort, advice and compassion. The leading way to convey that you are involved and compassionate about their key is to demonstrate that you are mentally there for them. Hand gestures, the position of the hands, and posture all convey interest in the exam.

Interaction over a camera should not be much different from interaction in person. While it is easy to get distracted or try to speed up the encounter by putting in orders or doing your notes while on with the patient, remember that it is a live interaction and that they are looking for your help.

Eye Contact

Eye contact is key in keeping both sides engaged in the encounter. The same as an in-person evaluation, eye contact allows the patient to feel that the provider is caring and engaged in the interaction. The adage *the eyes are the windows to the soul* rings true in this encounter. If the provider appears bored and their eyes are shifting around the screen, it sends the message that the patient is not important or that the provider would rather be somewhere else.

The focal point should be the camera and not the screen that the provider is working on. The camera would be the "eyes" of the patients while the screen would be their "body." It is OK to take your eyes off the camera and focus on the image on your screen periodically during the exam to look at a rash, in the throat, the digital assessment tools, or other facets of the evaluation.

The patient should overall feel focused upon, cared for, and welcome.

No Multitasking

Do not try to complete other tasks while on the telemedical encounter unless they are germane to the encounter at hand. Checking email, sorting through other patients' laboratory results, or other activities should not be completed during a telemedical evaluation. Looking at another screen that contains pertinent information, such as laboratory results, imaging results, consultant notes, and so on, is appropriate. Looking at personal information, social media, text messages, and email is not appropriate. The provider may think that the patient will never know what they are doing, but subtle clues are always present and decrease quality and satisfaction.

■ Communication

The provider must speak loud enough to be heard without yelling. However, the trick is that the patient should not feel they are being yelled at.

The language utilized during the evaluation is important. Support staff should recognize prior to the encounter if a translator is required or if any other services are needed. If proper accommodations cannot be met prior to the encounter, the patient should be invited to come in for an in-person evaluation.

■ Dress Code

The dress must remain professional. For many providers working from home, they have the option of a lax dress code. As healthcare professionals, we must remember our outward appearance is the first focus point for our patients.

Overall, nothing in this chapter should come as a surprise. Our patients want to feel cared for and heard. They should not walk away from a digital encounter wondering if the provider actually paid attention to them. This will harm their relationship not only with the provider but also with digital healthcare as a whole.

11

TECHNIQUES FOR ASSESSMENT AND PHYSICAL EXAM

▨ Introduction

Assessment by telemedicine and how to manipulate a physical exam completed by the patient are new concepts for all clinicians and patients. This is not only important for the assessment and diagnosis of the patient but for billing concerns as well.

Requirements for a patient-led physical exam include:

- ▨ Concise instructions
- ▨ Clear communications
- ▨ Verbal observations by the provider
- ▨ Kindness and understanding of the patients' concerns and fears

Remember to use nonmedical terms and language so patients and/or family members have a clear understanding of what you want them to perform. Using high-level medical language that cannot be easily understood frustrates and minimizes interaction. This leads to a decrease in the quality of the exam and distrust of the practitioner and the platform. A patient who would go to the emergency department because they did not trust the quality of a digital health examination defeats the purpose of that encounter and doubles the costs to the healthcare system. Remember, when coaching patients through an exam, the patient and/or family members completing this exam are sick, scared, and being asked to perform skills that they are not trained in.

▣ Step-by-Step

Use context clues and simple descriptions and take things markedly slower than if trained hands were performing the tasks. What you can observe, what is being described, and what hard data can be obtained (blood pressure, temperatures, glucose, pulse oximetry, heart rate) all help lead to a diagnosis or, at the very minimum, the ability to triage what can be addressed via digital health, what needs to be seen in the office, or what needs to be sent for emergent/urgent services.

Go back to where you were during nursing school or nurse practitioner training, medical school, or any other early form of education. How did you take information? Everything was slow and step-by-step. Everything was broken down into a system and data collected to be interpreted by a preceptor or senior provider.

Having the patient point, push, and move to the appropriate angle aids in the process. Use body landmarks that are easily found and avoid medical descriptions of the location (McBurney's point, Murphy's sign, etc.). The newer technology described in the remote patient monitoring section can aid in this evaluation process. However, this will not be mass-utilized as the majority of patients you will come across will not have this technology.

Overall, the assessment is similar to an in-person evaluation; the major difference is the patient or the person with the patient will be your hands.

▣ HEENT

Head

The shape of the head, any obvious injuries, and the texture of the hair all can carry clues to the provider. If the complaint is a headache, where and any corresponding skin changes can be noted and evaluated.

Ears

The presence of discharge, color of the skin, and exterior ear evaluations can be assessed. The interior ear evaluation can only be completed with specialized equipment that most patients will not have.

Eyes

The eye exam will be able to be completed via screen or family member. The presence of erythema, discharge, pupil shape, and size will not be able to be assessed by the patient without using a mirror or the front-facing camera on the phone (which the patient might be using for the evaluation). The ability of the eyes to focus on the provider can lead to other clues.

Nose

The nose exam can also be easily evaluated by the provider over the screen or if there is a second person present. Pay special attention to see if there are skin changes, erythema, discharge, or a foreign body present.

Throat

The throat cannot be evaluated by the patient without the use of other devices. The provider can attempt to evaluate the throat with or without the assistance of a second person. Erythema, discharge, exudate, swelling, and patency can be detected and utilized for diagnostic purposes.

Dental hygiene can also prove to be useful in assessing conditions of the mouth and oropharynx.

Having the patient utilize a flashlight to aid in the visualization of the nose and throat or having the friend or family member tell you what they can see will provide better quality information than trying to assess these over a screen.

Cardiopulmonary

Heart

You are most likely not going to be able to listen to heart sounds, but you will be able to assess rhythm, rate, and skin color/temperature. The patient or family member will be able to describe how the pulse feels, how fast it is, and if it is regular.

Lungs

Most patients you come across will not have stethoscopes. Therefore, lung sounds will not be assessable. The patient or family member should be able to count a respiratory rate and any audible sounds (wheezing, stridor). The patient's skin color and respiratory effort can also lead to valuable diagnostic clues.

The patient or family member may not say "wheezing" or "strider"; they may say a "teapot sound" or "squeaky sound."

Skin

This is the easiest system to evaluate by the provider over screen, the patient, or any family member. The temperature, texture, and presence of rash should all be noted. If there is a rash present, the characteristics of the rash can be described as well.

Abdomen

The abdominal exam can usually be completed by the patient themselves. However, a second person may increase the quality of the evaluation. The ability to identify if anything hurts with palpation, any obvious injuries, or abrasions.

Bowel sounds will most likely not be able to be assessed unless a stethoscope or other equipment is available.

Genitourinary

This assessment is the most difficult to assess as it will require the patient to be comfortable showing these areas over the screen. The presence of a significant other will aid in the evaluation of this area, to a degree. The patient can self-assess for the presence of masses, lesions or other abnormalities.

Musculoskeletal

This system is usually assessable via telemedicine. You will be able to see how the patient moves joints and muscle groups. It will be difficult to assess strength and discomfort against resistance unless there is a second person available to assist. The system might also require some movement of the camera angle as if you ask a person to move their arms while holding their phone or tablet, they might have to get creative with that device to allow the provider to visualize the requested movement.

Behavioral Health

This is probably the easiest to be evaluated over a digital platform. The ability to observe body language, speech patterns, and other diagnostic clues can be evaluated over the screen. Therapy can also be completed via telepsychiatry evaluations as this platform is perfect for a one-on-one conversation.

Following these tips should improve your physical exam no matter what body part is being assessed:

- Go slow.
- Be precise.
- Use common terminology, not medical.

- Ask for basic descriptors of what they are feeling.

- Use common language to describe specific sites for evaluation.

Remember, the one performing the physical exam is not a medical professional. They usually have no formal training, and they have something wrong with them. They can be feverish and nauseated, and they are likely scared and overwhelmed. The usual approach of going to the provider and letting them make all the assessments and interpretations is not there. Some patients may be completely new to the idea of digital health, and some may not understand even the simplest techniques. It is important not to get frustrated with the person on the other end of the computer as this will degrade everything you are trying to achieve.

To make everyone aware, there are great online resources that offer digital health assessment skills and have video examples on their website. This type of assessment comes with time, patience, and the ability to be creative and adapt.

REMOTE PATIENT MONITORING

Introduction

Remote patient monitoring (RPM) is a wonderful addition to the digital health arsenal. It allows for the patient and the provider to stay connected on their own schedules. Technology has allowed this gap to be bridged and providers to keep patients safe in an effective manner. From blood pressure (bp) monitors to scales to glucometers, the ability to monitor patients and transmit the data to the provider in real time provides a safety net for both parties. This information is then sent electronically to their provider or an agent thereof. Beginning January 1, 2018, Medicare allowed for billing of these services.

Case Example 1

A patient is recently discharge with a new diagnosis, new-onset atrial fibrillation with congestive heart failure (CHF) brought upon by uncontrolled bp and diabetes type 2. This patient is obese and lives with his wife; both are smokers. He is a retired factory worker and "quit" smoking 2 years ago, but he later admits to "sneaking one or two."

He was admitted to an acute care hospital for a week and then was transferred to a rehab facility for 2 weeks. In the acute care facility, he received serial laboratory evaluations, a cardiac catheterization, nutrition monitoring, and dietician support. He had daily weights, regular assessments of bp, heart rate, glucose, and heart rhythm. He was only placed on a low-sodium and fluid-restricted diet. He is now home on several new medications and has to complete follow-up exams with several specialists.

How can RPM help this patient? If this patient can be supplied with a dedicated telemedical team, which can include, but not be limited to, a nurse, a dietician, a social worker, a primary care provider (PCP), and specialty providers, his recovery and overall health status can greatly improve. Products such as bp monitors, portable electrocardiograms (EKGs), glucometers, scales, and devices that can be used to contact emergency services if required can be part of this patient's care plan. This patient may also benefit from close telehealth follow-ups from dieticians who can utilize a camera to see what the patient and wife keep in their kitchen and consider low sodium. A psychiatrist or psychologist can consult to assure he is coping with the new diagnosis as well as a physical therapist to assure he is staying mobile. Other members of the healthcare team can be brought in as needed.

▧ Patient Benefits of RPM

The new ability for patients to monitor themselves with real-time feedback from their provider increases compliance, adherence, and overall quality of care. If a patient's bp or glucose is consistently outside of a normal or acceptable range, they do not have to wait weeks to months for their follow-up appointment for correction of behaviors, medications or other factors. An intervention by the provider or auxiliary staff can be completed in a much timelier manner. Continuous glucose monitors that connect to the user's cellular phone as well as bp cuffs and other types of remote devices allow for this type of real-time feedback.

Availability of RPM

Everyday consumer products have become a more ready source of RPM. Apple, Google, and Fitbit watches and other similar products can monitor heart rate, hydration, steps, calories burned, activities, menstrual cycles, and a multitude of other health-monitoring processes. The Apple Watch specifically can call 911 automatically if an irregular and fast heart rate is noted or if a fall is detected. Scales can track weight and body mass index.

Medication Compliance and Adherence

Increased compliance with a treatment regimen increases the patient's overall health. If the patient does not take their meds as directed, they cannot have good health outcomes. To this end, RPM developers have created smart pill dispensers that allow for certain pills to be dispensed at their specific times. This replaces pillboxes or the common practice of a patient putting all their daily pills in one bottle. This also allows for the rapid identification of a patient's medication should an emergency situation arise.

Hospital at Home

The newer concept of "hospital at home," whereby low-risk hospitalizations can be monitored at home, is only possible via RPM. The ability to perform all the various point-of-care (POC) testing, including a troponin test and an electrocardiogram, is integral to this type of service. From there, the ability to complete a telecardiology evaluation from the PCP office is required to keep the care at an appropriate standard. The patient would then be sent home on a telemetry pack for overnight monitoring. This telemetry would be monitored by a qualified healthcare provider (paramedic, critical care nurse) and then repeat a POC troponin test in the morning with a follow-up telecardiology visit. Limiting factors would be family and personal history of heart disease, comorbid conditions, abnormal vital signs, or abnormal EKG. This is just one example of "hospital at home." This service decreases cost, increases satisfaction and, if proper emergency protocols are in place, serves as a safe, effect stand-in for the inpatient model of healthcare (see Appendix B for sample emergency protocols).

■ Case Example 2

Another example would be low-risk asthma or chronic obstructive pulmonary disorder exacerbation. This patient is evaluated, given intramuscular steroids, and completes a tele-pulmonologist visit. During the visit, the provider gives the patient a remote monitoring device with a pulse oximeter that directly sends information to a monitoring center and proper steroids, albuterol, and other medications. The next morning, the patient follows up with the PCP and the pulmonologist. The patient also receives social work and smoking cessation intervention in the hospital-at-home environment, as if they were admitted to an inpatient facility. Limiting factors for this scenario are hypoxemia (low blood oxygen), fever, the patient requiring oxygen, or comorbid conditions.

Both cases are limited by the availability of the equipment and monitoring services and coverage by the insurance company.

■ Monitoring Protocols

Every practice must have appropriate monitoring capabilities and protocols in place for both routine and emergency situations. Routine protocols include who qualifies for the hospital-at-home program, what medications should be provided and what to do if there is an emergency. Routine and emergency situations must all be solidified and easily accessible by the patient and the provider. Emergency protocols include the following:

- What would happen if an emergency occurred?
- Does the emergency services system get activated?
- Who activates the emergency system?
- How to approach monitoring the patient throughout the transfer of care process?

There are also payor-limiting factors, especially with government-based services (Medicare and Medicaid). This new way of managing patients outside of the hospital will save the system money and save acute care beds for patients who cannot meet the criteria for hospital-at-home services.

Drawbacks of RPM

Allowing the patient to be monitored at home requires appropriate technological infrastructure. Any organization that institutes RPM needs to assure access to the technology required. If the organization has a policy for hospital at home but does not have the equipment, it cannot perform those services.

Newer products on the market allow for complete evaluations to be completed at home, but they can be expensive. These products allow for home EKGs to be conducted and digital stethoscopes that allow for the provider to hear the heart, lungs, and bowel sounds in real time. These products also allow for visualization of the ears, nose, and throat. However, these products are not cheap, and that is part of the reason they are not widely used.

RPM is a very new addition to the digital health field of medicine, and many states do not pay for RPM services. This will change in time, and there is always the possibility that the COVID-19 pandemic will speed up these changes. We will know what effects COVID-19 will have on digital health and specifically RPM in time. The advancement of RPM and its availability will continue to allow this type of service to become mainstream.

IV

COVID-19 AND TELEMEDICINE

13

COVID-19 RESPONSE TO TELEMEDICINE AND LESSONS LEARNED

▨ Converting to Telemedicine During COVID-19

During the COVID-19 pandemic the world shut down. Most care delivery organizations (CDOs) were forced to come up with emergent digital health options for treating their patients. These responses, no matter what stage of digital health planning the CDO was in prior to March 2020, were thrust into high gear, and digital health was pushed to the front-burner.

Setting up a completely online medical practice from a traditional brick-and-mortar one was not an easy task in the middle of a pandemic, especially if the practice contains multi specialties and a patient and provider population not familiar with the concept of telemedicine. The intricacies of involving specialty care, including surgical specialists, required time and consideration that many practices did not have. As a result, appropriate care methods and workflows were revisited on multiple occasions.

Staff and providers needed to rapidly learn the intricacies of a digital health evaluation and how to manage patients via this platform. Education was vital, on how to schedule, when to find an in-person provider and how to properly prescribe for these patients. The constantly changing laws from the governors of the state, the Centers for Medicare and Medicaid Services (CMS), and the federal government made this especially challenging.

During the height of the COVID-19 pandemic, hospital beds, especially monitored and vent-capable beds and units, were at a premium. Long-term acute care hospitals and intensive care units were full, and overflow units were pushed to their breaking point. Keeping patients healthy, limiting the spread of COVID-19, and preventing worsening chronic diseases were the goals of digital health during this time. Imagine if more digital health capabilities were in place, especially in the area of remote patient monitoring. With more widespread remote monitoring equipment, especially the products that offer the ability for providers to monitor patients in real time, more patients could have been quarantined at home.

■ Legislative Changes During COVID-19

At the legislative level, several laws were adjusted at the federal and state levels to allow for the greater availability of digital health options.

Commercial platforms such as WhatsApp, Skype, Face-Time and Facebook Messenger were allowed for digital health services by the CMS. Others like Zoom and Cisco WebEx became especially popular in all aspects, not just digital health services.

Hierarchical condition category (HCC) codes were allowed to be billed via telemedicine and the associated attestation forms completed. This utilized the real-time audio/video synchronous telemedical approach. Wellness exams could also be billed via real-time audio/video services; however, this was difficult to implement with limited to no ability to perform a physical evaluation except for what the patient could do to themselves.

Copays and coinsurance were also waived or reduced when the visit was related to COVID-19. The eligibility of providers such as physical and occupational therapists, speech and language pathologists and others were able to bill for Medicare digital health services. Inpatient billing for telemedical services was also increased by the CMS during COVID-19.

The Drug Enforcement Agency (DEA) also relaxed some of itsprovisions, especially with regard to Schedule 2 Controlled Dangerous Substances (CDSs). It allowed Schedule 2 medications to be called in for a short "emergency supply" (about a 3 days' supply).

Providers of all licensures were freed to care for patients across state lines. Collaborative and/or supervisory agreements between nurse practitioners or physician assistants to supervising and collaborating physicians were removed. The rules governing this waiver in the CMS guidelines stated that the provider must be enrolled in Medicare, possess a valid license, provide services in a state where a state of emergency exists, and not be barred from practice in the state where services are being provided. Some states also offered to allow clinicians to provide care only if they were not planning on opening a physical location.

The following table demonstrates some of the laws that were modified, stopped, or otherwise altered to provide telemedical care during the COVID-19 pandemic. The information is from the Federation of State Medical Boards. The information is for guidance only as the organization should go to the source for full information.

A disproportionate amount of legislation relates to physicians versus advanced practice clinician (APC) professionals. This may be because many states require APCs to practice under physicians in one form or another. All APCs should consult the state practice guides prior to performing telemedical services. It is also clear that most legislative changes regarded services covered, the elimination of state border licensure requirements, and CDS prescriptive procedures.

TABLE 13.1 **STATE LEGISLATION CHANGES DUE TO COVID-19**

State	Changes	Source
Alabama	Physicians from other states can provide telemedical services	ALBME Telemedicine Guidance
	Temporary emergency medical licenses can be received	State Resource page
Alaska	Providers can diagnosis and prescribe without an in-person evaluation first	AK SB 241
	Providers could issue CDS prescriptions without an in-person evaluation	Emergency Regulations
	Opioid medication treatments can be done without in-person evaluations	Bulletin 20-07 Re: Telehealth Coverage
Arizona	Temporary MD and DO licenses could be provided	AMB Guidance
	Governor ordered insurance companies to pay for tele-medical services	Executive Order (EO) 2020-15
	Department of Health is not allowed to prohibit, investigate, and take action again licensed health professionals with regard to price gouging during COVID	Executive Order (EO) 2020-07

(continued)

TABLE 13.1 **STATE LEGISLATION CHANGES DUE TO COVID-19 (*CONTINUED*)**

State	Changes	Source
Arkansas	EO 20-16 allows physicians from TX, OK, MO, TN, MI, and LA privileges to perform telemedical services for established patients	Border State Emergency License
	No need for in-person evaluations prior to telemedical services	EO 20-16
	CDS can be prescribed for 6 months as long it is a refill and not a new prescription	EO 20-05
		Telemedicine Guidance
California	Government code section 179.5 allows for medical services to be provided in California	Emergency Declaration
	Out-of-state medical personnel submits requests to EMS authority and sign "request for temporary recognition of out of state medical personnel during a state of emergency"	EMSA Guidance
	EO N-43-20 enabled protections to medical providers for telemedical services for exposure to COVID-19	Temporary License Application

(*continued*)

TABLE 13.1 **STATE LEGISLATION CHANGES DUE TO COVID-19 (*CONTINUED*)**

State	Changes	Source
	Eliminates need for provider to obtain verbal/written consent before the use of telehealth services and document same	EO N-43-20
Colorado	A physician can provide services in CO as long as the service is gratuitous without restrictions	DORA Guidance
	Patients are not required to be in the state of CO	
Connecticut	Suspends licensure requirements which establishes who may qualify as a "telemedical provider"	EO 7G
	Department of public health may establish a process of allowing out-of-state applicant medical license	Conn. Gen. Stat. 20-12
	Waives the homebound requirements for new patient telemedical evaluations	CMAP Telemedicine Guidance
Delaware	Health care professionals who have active licenses in good standing allowed to provide in-person care in DE during COVID-19	DEMA/DPH Order

(continued)

TABLE 13.1 **STATE LEGISLATION CHANGES DUE TO COVID-19 (*CONTINUED*)**

State	Changes	Source
	Mental health providers can provide in-person and tele-medicine services	Medical Board Reg. 19
	All in-person requirements related to telemedicine services under state title 24 is waived	
Florida	EO for certain out-of-state healthcare providers to allow for telemedical services	DOH EO 20-002
	Health care providers can provide services for a period up to 30 days if they have a valid medical license	DOH EO 20-003
	Renewal prescriptions for CDS can be provided	DOH EO 20-004
	Out-of-state practitioners can perform telehealth services and must register with the medical board of Florida	FL DOH Guidance
		2019-137
Georgia	Emergency practice permits to out-of-state licensed professionals	GA Code 43-34-31.1

(continued)

TABLE 13.1 **STATE LEGISLATION CHANGES DUE TO COVID-19 (*CONTINUED*)**

State	Changes	Source
	Telemedical licenses can be provided to out-of-state licenses	Emergency Practice Applications
	Electronic CDS prescriptions without in-person medical evaluations	
Hawaii	Suspended Section 453-1.3 allows for out-of-state telehealth services without in-person care	EO 20-02
Idaho	Out-of-state physicians and PAs with a license in good standing do not need an Idaho license to practice telemedicine during COVID-19	Idaho Telehealth Act
	Suspension of telehealth access 54-5705 regarding preexisting provider/patient relationship with regard to CDS	EO 20-13
	Allows use of Zoom, FaceTime, and others to practice telemedicine	
	EO for out-of-state providers to practice telemedicine	

(continued)

TABLE 13.1 **STATE LEGISLATION CHANGES DUE TO COVID-19 (CONTINUED)**

State	Changes	Source
Illinois	EO 2020-9 allows for out-of-state health care providers to provide services	EO 2020-09
	Telehealth services expanded to all providers and can utilize FaceTime, Facebook Messenger, Google Hangouts, or Skype	Articles Re: Telehealth and Origination Site
	Payors cannot impose utilization review requirements or prior authorization requirements and must cover costs of telehealth services	
Indiana	EO 20-05 eliminated requirement of an in-state license if there is a license held in another state	EO 20-05
	Initial Telemedicine Provider Certification Request must be completed first and prescriptive privileges are based on IC 25-1-9.5-8	PLA Guidance
	Mental health workers can function via telemedicine	IC 250109.5-8
	Chronic pain CDS can be prescribed via audio-only and audio/visual telemedicine	EO 20-13

(continued)

TABLE 13.1 **STATE LEGISLATION CHANGES DUE TO COVID-19 (*CONTINUED*)**

State	Changes	Source
Iowa	Physician may practice without a state license IF licensedin another state	Board of Med Emergency Declaration 3/16 and 4/27
	All previously established rules for telemedicine/telehealth services are suspended	EO 3/24
	CDS would not require face-to-face evaluations	
Kansas	EO to expand use of telemedicine and waive restrictions on providers from out of state	EO 20-08
	Every physician treating patients via telemedicine should conduct an appropriate assessment and evaluation and document appropriately	
Kentucky	MD/DO may register to practice within Kentucky during COVID	KBML Guidance
	KY SB 150 waives requirements of in-person exams	KY SB 150

(*continued*)

TABLE 13.1 **STATE LEGISLATION CHANGES DUE TO COVID-19 (*CONTINUED*)**

State	Changes	Source
	1915© HCBC (Medicaid) waivers for out-of-state licenses providers	
	Services can be completed via phone and telemedicine	
Louisiana	Emergency temporary permit for out-of-state medical professionals	LSBME Telemedicine Permits
	CDS can be prescribed	Proclamation 2020-32
	Must use a secure HIPAA compliant server but can use commercial services if no other option is available	LDH Guidance 3/20
	No limitations on originating site	Telehealth Guidance
Maine	MD/DO/PA/NP can provide out-of-state services	Supplemental Order 3/20
	Maximize use of telemedicine and telehealth to eliminate the need for in-person evaluations	EO 3/24

(continued)

TABLE 13.1 **STATE LEGISLATION CHANGES DUE TO COVID-19 (*CONTINUED*)**

State	Changes	Source
Maryland	SB 1080 authorized governor to establish or waive telehealth protocols for COVID-19 including usage of out-of-state professionals to provide continuity of care	Maryland SB 1080
	CDS requires MD CDS registration to prescribe	Notice Re: CDS 5/8
	The link for telemedical services must be secure and private	EO 4/1
	CDS can be prescribed	
	Governor allowed for all providers to use telemedical services and can utilize audio-only calls	
Massachusetts	Temporary licensure for out-of-state professionals	BORIM Press Release
	No in-person evaluation requirements	Article Re: Preexisting Relationship Rrequirements
	Payors must reimburse same rate as in-person care	Article. Re: Coverage

(*continued*)

TABLE 13.1 **STATE LEGISLATION CHANGES DUE TO COVID-19 (*CONTINUED*)**

State	Changes	Source
	Doctor on Demand drafted by state legislature to provide free services for self-pay patients	Article Re: Uninsured
Michigan	Encouraged use of telemedical or telehealth services	LARA Clarification
	Allows for out-of-state providers	EO 2020-86
	Written consent not required	
	RPM can be used	
	CDS can be prescribed without in-person evaluation	
Minnesota	Allows for out-of-state providers for telemedical services, includes behavioral health providers	EO 20-46
	CMS allowed for data collection from out-of-state providers	MN Statute 147.032
	More than three telemedical visits can be completed for medical assistance	EO 20-29

(*continued*)

TABLE 13.1 **STATE LEGISLATION CHANGES DUE TO COVID-19 (*CONTINUED*)**

State	Changes	Source
	Expands the definition of telemedicine to include phone calls for providers with an agreement with the Minnesota Department of Health	Article Re: Medicaid/ Waiver
Mississippi	If a physician's specialty is required, an out-of-state license may be issued	Supplemental Proclamation 4/5
	Preexisting doctor–patient relationships doesn't apply for in-state physicians	Amended Proclamation 3/24
Missouri	Physicians and surgeons licensed in another state can care for Missouri citizens in person on telemedicine	EO 20-04
	EO suspends rules requiring a physical exam	Article Re: Telehealth
Montana	Provides interstate licensure when needed by a state of emergency. Strict requirements of telehealth practitioners are suspended	EO MCA 10-3-118
	Telemedicine or telehealth can utilize all platforms	Gubernatorial Directive 4/21

(continued)

TABLE 13.1 **STATE LEGISLATION CHANGES DUE TO COVID-19 (*CONTINUED*)**

State	Changes	Source
	Telemedicine coverage much be the same as in-person care	
Nebraska	Health care providers not required to obtain a patient's signature for telehealth consent	DHHS Guidance
		EO 20-10
Nevada	Allows for reinstitution of medical licenses due to not completing CMEs, those who have retired, and out-of-state medical licenses	Emergency Directive 011
New Hampshire	Out-of-state medical providers can perform necessary services	EO #15
	Telehealth could perform services via all modalities	EO #8
	Payors must reimburse for telemedical services as they would for in-person	EO #29
	CDS can be prescribed via telemedicine	Board of Mental Health Practice Guidance

(continued)

TABLE 13.1 **STATE LEGISLATION CHANGES DUE TO COVID-19 (*CONTINUED*)**

State	Changes	Source
	Telemental services can perform out-of-state care	
New Jersey	NJ will waive several regulatory requirements including those related to telemedicine and telehealth	AG Guidance
	Payors must allow their customers about telemedical services	Telehealth Insurance Bulletin 3/10
New Mexico	NM shall allow out-of-state providers to render necessary services; NM Stat 12-10-11	NM Stat 12-10-11
	Electronic means to assess and provide care will not be unethical or violation of medical board rules	NMMB Guidance
New York	Out-of-state licensed providers will be allowed to serve population of NY	EO 202.5
	Section 596 of title 14 can allow for rapid approval of telemental services	EO 202

(*continued*)

TABLE 13.1 **STATE LEGISLATION CHANGES DUE TO COVID-19 (*CONTINUED*)**

State	Changes	Source
	Insurance company to waive copay related to COVID	Statement on Co-Pay Waived 3/14
	Telephone, telehealth, and telemedical services should be encouraged	NYC Health Advisory
North Carolina	Section 16 of EO 116 allows for out-of-state providers to practice	EO 130
	BC BS of NC will cover tele-medical visits	EO 116
		Article Re: Reimbursement
North Dakota	Behavioral health professionals and physicians/surgeons can provide out-of-state care	EO 2020-05.1
	Insurance carrier will cover virtual check-ins	
Ohio	Code 4731.36 will allow out-of-state telemedicine for physicians treating patients visiting OH and physicians in contiguous states can provide care	Board of Med 4/20

(*continued*)

TABLE 13.1 **STATE LEGISLATION CHANGES DUE TO COVID-19 (*CONTINUED*)**

State	Changes	Source
	Suspend enforcement of in-person first exams	Ohio Rev. Code 4731.36'
	Telemedicine can be used in place of in-person exams	
	Allows for CDS prescriptions	
Oklahoma	Out-of-state providers can practice in OK	Amended EO 2020-07
	Telemedicine and telehealth can be allowed to provide care for new and existing services	COVID-19 Pandemic Emergency Rules
	No existing doctor–patient is required for CDS	Article Re: Preexisting Relationship
Oregon	Physicians and PAs can practice from out of state	Board of Med Guidance
	CDS cannot be prescribed by an out-of-state provider	Emergency Application
	Out-of-state physicians cannot act as a supervising physician of EMTs or PAs	

(continued)

TABLE 13.1 **STATE LEGISLATION CHANGES DUE TO COVID-19 (*CONTINUED*)**

State	Changes	Source
Pennsylvania	Out-of-state licensed professionals are allowed for a telemedical service	Press Release
		PA Dept. of State Guidance
Rhode Island	Encouraging telemedical services	EO 20-06
	Patients may receive telemedical services at any location	RIDOH Guidance
	Clinically appropriate medically necessary telemedicine services should be reimbursed at the same rate as in-person evaluations	Press Release Re: Coverage
South Carolina	Out-of-state licensed professionals are allowed	Article Re: OOS Licensure
	CDS of Schedule 2 and 3 medications can be provided via telemedicine	BME Order
		EO 2020-BME-PH-03

(*continued*)

TABLE 13.1 **STATE LEGISLATION CHANGES DUE TO COVID-19 (*CONTINUED*)**

State	Changes	Source
South Dakota	Compact state members can provide in-person care or remote means	EO 2020-07
	Regulations were eliminated regarding telemedicine or telehealth services	
Tennessee	Out-of-state providers can complete telemedical services	Article: OOS License
	Telehealth with regard to pain management is suspended	EO 15
	Masters or doctoral degree in behavioral or mental health field can diagnosis and treat without a license	EO 20
	BC BS of TN will cover virtual visits	EO 24
Texas	Out-of-state in-person and telemedical providers allowed	TMB Guidance 5/8
	Refill of CDS with established relationships	TMB Guidance 6/5

(continued)

TABLE 13.1 **STATE LEGISLATION CHANGES DUE TO COVID-19 (*CONTINUED*)**

State	Changes	Source
	Audio-only telemedicine encounters allowed	Article Re: Telemedicine
	Written or oral consent must be obtained	Governor's Press Release
Utah	Out-of-state physicians may practice	UT Code Annotated 58-67-305(7)
	Providers must alert patients if they are not using HIPAA or HITECH compliant platforms	
Vermont	Physicians, PAs, and podiatrists can practice in VT if their services are emergent and necessary and free to the patients	Med Board Guidance
	Must have an active out-of-state license	Deemed License Application
Virginia	Out-of-state licensed professionals will be allowed to provide continuity of care to current patients	Board of Medicine Guidance

(*continued*)

TABLE 13.1 **STATE LEGISLATION CHANGES DUE TO COVID-19 (*CONTINUED*)**

State	Changes	Source
	Healthcare practitioner may use non-public-facing audio or remote communication whether the diagnosis is COVID or something else	EO 42
		EO 57
Washington	Volunteer out-of-state providers will be allowed and can apply for expedited licensure	Medical Commission Guidance
	Parity laws instituted to allow for the same reimbursement for telemedical/telehealth as in-person care	Emergency Volunteer Health Practitioners
		Emergency Proclamation 20-29
		RCW 70.15.050
Washington D.C.	Out-of-state providers licensed in their home state will be agents of the District and allowed to perform services via telehealth if the provider has an existing relationship	Waiver of Licensure Requirements

(*continued*)

TABLE 13.1 **STATE LEGISLATION CHANGES DUE TO COVID-19 (*CONTINUED*)**

State	Changes	Source
	Out-of-state providers will require a D.C. license	Guidance on Use of Tele-Medicine
		DC Code 3-1205.02
West Virginia	Suspension of requirements for telemedicine providers to be licensed in WV if provider has a license in their home state	EO 07-20
	WV expanded use of audio/video telehealth for none-mergent services	
Wisconsin	Physician providing telemedicine must have a license issued by this state, another state, or Canada without restrictions	EO 16
Wyoming	Physicians and PAs can work in WY under a consulting exemption	Board of Med Guidance
	They will be consultants with the State Health Officer	Emergency Licensure Application

(*continued*)

TABLE 13.1 **STATE LEGISLATION CHANGES DUE TO COVID-19 (CONTINUED)**

State	Changes	Source
	Once the physician has been approved for the consultation exemption, they may generate new patients	
	Telehealth technology must allow to meet standard of care	

AG, attorney general; ALBME, Alabama Board of Medical Examiners; AMB, Arizona Medical Board; BORIM, Board of Registration in Medicine; CDS, Controlled Dangerous Substances; CMAP, Connecticut Medical Assistance Program; CMS, Centers for Medicare and Medicaid Services; DEMA, Delaware Emergency Management Agency; DHHS, Department of Health and Human Services; DO, doctors of osteopathy; DPH, Division of Public Health; EMS, emergency medical services; EMSA, Emergency Medical Services Authority; EMTs, emergency medical technicians; HCBC, home and community-based services; HIPAA, Health Information Privacy and Portability Act; HITECH, Health Information Technology for Economic and Clinical Health; KBML, Kentucky Board of Medical Licensure; LARA, Licensing and Regulatory Affairs; LDH, Louisiana Department of Health; LSBME, Louisiana State Board of Medical Examiners; MD, medical doctors; NMMB, New Mexico Medical Board; NP, Nurse Practitioners; OOS, office online server; PA, physician assistant; PLA, professional licensing agency; RIDOH, Rhode Island Department of Health; RPM, remote patient monitoring.

COVID-19 was one of the darkest hours in history. The availability of current technology both for the digital medical world and the general digital world makes this pandemic markedly different from previous ones. Revoking constrictive rules and regulations by the legislators (the president, Congress, and governors) and payors (the CMS and commercial) increased access to care and allowed providers to get appropriately compensated for their services. The hope for digital health is that post-COVID, legislators see the benefits of this field of medicine and allow it to blossom and grow.

14

DIGITAL HEALTH FOR EDUCATION AND FAMILY SUPPORT

▓ Digital Health in Education

For the past several years, education has been going online, allowing flexibility for students who need to work, meet childcare obligations, or perform other tasks to still get an education. This was enhanced starting March 2020. When the global pandemic of COVID-19 hit, schools were forced to close their doors. This included medical, nursing, and other allied healthcare providers receiving their last rounds of education before graduating electronically. Continuing education, cardiopulmonary resuscitation training, and even some board testing became a remote operation. The readily available technology opened a door that had been closed by the public health emergency of COVID-19.

During the height of the COVID-19 public health emergency, schools of all levels were forced to go to a digital method of education. While the mainstream media portrayed this as a new development, digital education has been in effect for many years. The largest difference between now and then is the sheer number of those going through online education.

The ability of the schools to open their doors to more students while using fewer brick-and-mortar resources seems to be a solution for lowering their costs and keeping the costs that are then translated to students down. That being said, there are always going to be situations in which in-person education must remain (clinical laboratories, science laboratories, and acting and performance art programs all come to mind).

Digital health has also allowed the ability to renew certifications, licenses, and other professional credentials electronically. This increases compliance and ease of completing these tasks. With the past providers, staff and students would have had to take days off work and school to complete these tasks; webcams and other creative techniques allow for sufficient measuring and evaluation of the candidate.

Electronic education has been evolving and growing. There has become a new standard that all conferences, continuing education, and intraoffice meetings have become web-based. While this may not be a new feature of most environments, it has certainly never been the mainstay it has become.

Professional conferences have also begun going to an electronic format out of necessity. Starting in the spring of 2021, these conferences, which throughout 2020 were purely electronic, became hybrid. This allowed for those who were willing and able to attend in person to do so while those who were unable or unwilling to still participate. The increased availability and decreased expense of a virtual conference will certainly be a huge draw for more participants to attend. While information sharing is still available, the majority of people go to these conferences for networking and other social aspects that are lost via internet-based platforms. However, new and developing mediums currently allow, and will going forward, more personal interactions.

▨ Digital Health for Family Support

The ability to communicate via portable electronic means has changed our society greatly over the last few years. Vast amounts of communication occur over commercial audio and visual means such as FaceTime, Google Hangouts, Skype, or a myriad of other platforms. This has changed the dynamic of communication and allows for direct access to their friends and loved ones.

During the COVID-19 pandemic, it wasn't uncommon for loved ones to say good-bye over a screen. There were several articles about nurses and other healthcare professionals using their own devices to FaceTime or utilize another video chat program for families to talk one last time before a patient going on a respirator or expiring. Travel during COVID was also significantly limited. For many families who needed to check in on children or elderly parents, technology was the only way to accommodate this.

The sadness of COVID-19 allowed for periods of kindness and once again demonstrates the vast abilities of healthcare professionals to provide social care to the patients in their charge. Due to infection control measures being implemented, families were forced to leave loved ones at the entrance to the hospital with the hope of seeing them again.

Digital health and the use of electronics for family support and communication is here to stay. With hope, time, and science, we will no longer have to use this medium to say good-bye to a loved one but rather keep them informed and offer a method for staying current on healthcare.

Family Education

How families interact and engage with the healthcare system is changing and evolving. It used to be taboo to instruct your patients to utilize YouTube or other nonmedical websites to gather information. During the COVID-19 pandemic, especially in the early days of the public health emergency, it was common to utilize YouTube videos for yoga, Pilates, or similar for muscle pains in the place of physical therapy. Many products also offer links via electronic means or Quick Response codes directly to YouTube or Vimeo, where they have stored demonstration videos for application or usage of their products.

Patients and families are also utilizing phone applications or websites to get nutrition information, ask questions of technical staff or nurses, and watch product demonstrations. While those who need specialized healthcare-related information should defer to licensed providers, nutritionists, and other specialties, the public can utilize these services for safe and effective modifications to diet and exercise.

Telehealth platforms, including commercial platforms such as Zoom, have also become popular when providing patient education. Especially in the days of COVID, it was not feasible to spend prolonged periods in an enclosed area with another person or group of people. Education that used to take place in person is now occurring over electronic means. The ability to incorporate different languages, sign language interpreters, and other translation means allow providers and patients alike to participate with ease.

Overall, as demonstrated elsewhere in this book, the electronic transmission of data and education is now the common means of relaying information. Most people, in fact, seem to enjoy the at-home, self-paced electronic education as they can reference as needed and go at their own pace. This is likely to continue post-COVID and grow in popularity. Online, interactive means is an area likely to grow and become more functional, which will only increase its popularity.

15

MY TELEMEDICINE STORY AND THE FUTURE OF DIGITAL HEALTH

◼ My Telemedicine Story

In 2015, my employer and I started the general discussion about applying a digital health solution to the practice. We met to discuss the needs, risks, and benefits of telemedicine. Limiting factors at the time were the cost, functionality, availability, and reimbursement. These discussions took place before the parity law passed in New Jersey regarding equal pay for telemedical services in 2017.

After several years with endless calls and emails to potential vendors, some never making it past phone calls and PowerPoint presentations, we tried our first platform. This was a success in that the platform was functional and available. It was a failure in that the reimbursement and interest were just not there. Between these trials and discussions with vendors, I researched the telemedicine approaches, laws, platforms, and the Centers for Medicare and Medicaid Services (CMS) recommendations regarding digital health. When we began to coordinate efforts with our sister organization, the digital health platform started to take off.

We started working with this company, partnering on cost and productivity and negotiating a contract that would benefit both sides equally while maximizing the utilization of the product. After having several meetings regarding this platform, we were given the go-ahead from the executive team. We established platform negotiations and timelines and formalized the creation team.

The week of March 9, 2020, was a blur. We had numerous meetings, in person and virtually, for the application of digital health on the coming pandemic. Each day of that week we discussed ideas for different platforms, including an emergency version of the platform we had planned on using long term. None of these solutions made it past the planning and discussion stage.

Thursday morning, we settled on a commercial platform, WhatsApp, and I worked with our chief medical officer (CMO), chief operations officer (COO), and chief executive officer (CEO) as well as the president and founder of the practice to bring this platform online in 24 hours. We rushed to acquire proper equipment and create workflows that would meet the needs of the practice and a population in turmoil. That night, we were told we could not utilize the commercial platform and found another more secure application that our psychiatric department had utilized with some success.

The next day, coincidentally Friday the 13th, was supposed to be my day off. Instead, it turned into a day full of workflow discussions, billing codes, utilization management, and video and conference calls with the platform. I needed privileges to access the system, and then I needed additional platform privileges for electronic prescription and Controlled Dangerous Substances. While I went through provider training, the administrator and auxiliary staff also required their logins and training.

Monday, we went live. We had constant workflow adjustments, noted the need for additional staff, and had to sort out who qualified for COVID-19 testing and who needed to monitor symptoms for 2 to 3 days before testing because of limited supplies for testing. We saw 30 patients that day and 60 patients the next. By the end of the week, with a load of 250 patients, we recruited the CEO and the CMO to help with calls and find other providers to pick up the overflow of patients. The support team increased from 2 to 3 people to about 15 to 20 members. By the next Monday, many of our offices were closed, and we essentially went to a 95% telemedical practice. The specialists in our group started performing telemedical services as well.

My practice went through several iterations and platforms in a very short period. Working through workflow with platform information technology (IT) professionals, salespeople, and software engineers to have their programs meet their needs proved unsuccessful in the first several attempts. During the first few weeks of the telemedical services during COVID-19, we switched to Zoom and utilized its base form with a business associate agreement . We eventually changed again, moving up to the healthcare version of that platform.

We utilized different telehealth approaches during the COVID-19 pandemic as well. During that initial week, between patients, I helped with the support calls to introduce telemedicine and assessment techniques to the providers. Setting up the basis to care for more than 5,000 telemedical visits a day during the height of the pandemic took some doing.

For the providers and medical assistant staff, we had to properly educate how to do telemedical assessments:

- Visual assessments
- Relying on history
- Patient self-assessments or family assessments
- Utilizing phone applications or home medical devices
- Proper billing and coding techniques

The medical reception staff needed to learn about who paid or didn't have to pay copays or coinsurances. There were many changing rules and regulations regarding payment structures. This changed on a daily or weekly basis.

Throughout the pandemic, we had educational meetings with the providers completed by our CEO, CMO, CPO (chief pediatric officer), and CNO (chief nursing officer). Digital platforms such as Zoom and Citrix Webex were utilized for all meetings that were usually completed in person.

We utilized remote patient monitoring (RPM) during the COVID crisis as patients were forced home. For patients with COVID-19 who reported shortness of breath, we asked them to monitor their oxygen level and heart rate with devices they could purchase online or smartphone applications. While these were not the first choice, they became valuable tools for monitoring patients from home with close follow-ups via telemedicine to assess if the patient needed further care with our pulmonologist, home oxygen, or emergency care and possible admission to an inpatient facility. We also prescribed more blood pressure cuffs and glucometers than before as we requested patients to monitor these metrics for themselves instead of coming to the office for these evaluations.

Overall, COVID-19 launched our digital health platform in a way that I could never have imagined. We realized the abilities of the cyber world could be effectively applied to the medical world and allowed us to continue high-quality care to our patients. Overall, we saw more than 100,000 patients in 3 months with great success and minimal concerns with its application. How far it will go and what our digital footprint will be going forward are yet to be seen.

■ The Future of Digital Health

The future of digital health is unlimited. As long as the technology continues to advance, so will telemedicine and digital health. Every aspect of our lives depends on technology; healthcare should be no different. If we can turn our homes into smart homes, why can't we turn our healthcare smart as well? The most important factors in the advancement of digital health are that the technology be affordable, the software be accessible, and the providers be kind, compassionate, and have knowledge of the application of telemedicine and RPM. The technology will always advance, and the CMS and commercial payors will eventually catch up to the requested services.

The ability of a patient's healthcare to have real-time interactions and reply in a dynamic and potentially lifesaving manner is paramount. RPM and hospital at home allow for patients to stay out of the hospital unless they are in critical condition. This not only decreases the cost to the healthcare system and potential exposure to other conditions or diseases, but it also increases the quality and comfort of the care. The benefits to the patient are also limitless as the desire and technology continue to advance.

Decreasing the use of expensive resources and increasing high-tech, low-cost avenues of healthcare will lead to an improved overall healthcare system. When patients' poor decisions can be modified in real time, this allows for immediate intervention to prevent worsening health and the development of comorbidities. Coaching for smoking cessation, drug and alcohol rehabs, and pregnancy and childrearing support are slowly but surely being developed for the benefit of all.

A video game named *Endeavor RX* was recently released for the treatment of attention-deficit hyperactivity disorder for children. Software platforms such as this can be implemented by therapists, primary care providers, and specialists to decrease the cost of the healthcare system, decrease the frequency of visits, decrease the usage of potentially harmful pharmaceuticals, and allow for care to be provided from the comfort of their home.

The digital health platform can also monitor the safety and satisfaction of the providers and staff. As illuminated by the recent COVID-19 pandemic, provider burnout can occur very quickly with disastrous results. Some providers feel guilty, embarrassed, or isolated seeking care themselves as they are the ones who are supposed to be providing this service. With digital health, they can be screened, seek mental health services, and receive care. For COVID-19 specifically, mobile apps can check risk factors or symptoms such as cough, shortness of breath, and fever prior to reporting for your shift. If any symptoms are present, the app can direct you where to go and who to alert.

Involving emergency medical services (EMS) in a digital health solution is a newer aspect of this care platform. Since the mid-1900s paramedics have used radios or telephone to describe a situation and relay pertinent facts to the emergency department (ED) physician so medical orders can be carried out prior to the paramedics' arrival to the ED. For example, paramedics can transmit the image of the vital signs and an electrocardiogram (EKG) to the physician. In the case of a potential heart attack, this could activate the team and decrease the door to balloon time (heart catheterization).

What other aspects of EMS services could be influenced by digital health? Some states have placed nurse practitioners (NPs) or physician assistants (PAs) on paramedic ambulances, allowing for community outreach, more appropriate utilization of emergency resources, and decongestion of ED volume. This could be further revolutionized by allowing NPs or PAs to work remotely and have access to a higher volume of patients. Patients who call 911 for medication refills, simple upper respiratory infections, minor injuries, and all types of low-risk urgent, but not emergent, situations could be cared for at home instead of clogging up the ED.

Applications that help monitor weight, activity, smoking, and other metrics of a patient's health also allow for these conditions to be monitored more closely. Everyone likes games and movies. If the intervention entertaining and metric tracking does not feel like work, the patient will be more compliant. If the devices will monitor their vitals, glucose or other factors and send this information directly to the providers, the middleman of the patient gets removed.

There will always be a future for digital health services. Technology is one of the fastest moving modalities in our society, and it is time to harness this for healthcare. Using COVID-19 to push forth the digital health applications to standing organizations and chief data officers, we can modify emergency responses systems put in place to a long-standing digital health platform. As technology advances and products, applications, and software become more available, the future of digital health is limitless.

■ Conclusion

Digital health and telemedicine are here to stay. How we use them currently and how we develop them are the only variables. With proper support and cultivation, we can elevate this aspect of our care to the next level. This will provide an even higher level of care for our patient population and, in the world of risk-based medicine, an increased profit for digital health–equipped practices.

While the history of telemedicine has vast roots, the future is far from written. The advance of available technology has grown exponentially in recent years and can only be expected to grow further going forward. With smart devices penetrating every aspect of our lives, it is not hard to see how digital health can become part of mainstream healthcare.

COVID-19 has taught the medical community and their consumers much about digital health, telemedicine, and RPM. It is the job of everyone involved to not forget the lessons of the past, as *those who do not study history are doomed to repeat it*. The lessons learned during the global pandemic of 2020 will allow the digital health practitioners of the future to flourish.

Laws, rules, and regulations will continue to change. There is always a lag between the law and the technology to support it. The innovative provider will assure that, while they may be constrained by the laws of the state, they continue to provide the highest quality care via a digital medium.

Providers that become comfortable and proficient in telemedicine and telehealth must teach future generations of providers. Administrators must do the same with auxiliary staff, and the patient outreach teams should continue to work on more effective ways of communicating with patients. Workflow will always ensure the smoothest and most efficient care of the patient. Everyone must share the lessons learned.

Where we go with digital health is unknown, but it will always be part of the package of healthcare. It will continue to evolve and create more abilities to care for patients outside of a brick-and-mortar location.

APPENDICES

APPENDIX A: CASE STUDY: MM

MM is a 51-year-old male patient who came to see me for the first time to evaluate why he was feeling fatigued, had a dry mouth, and was always thirsty and urinating to excess. He had a history of diabetes but never took medication. His glucose registered as "HI" with 2+ glucose and 1+ ketones in the urine but as he had no other complaints and his physical exam was normal; he was sent home after blood was collected for laboratory analysis. This patient refused being sent to the emergency room for these symptoms.

He returned the next day to be reevaluated and discuss the laboratory tests. His pertinent results were as follows:

Glucose: 654 mg/dL
Sodium: 126 mg/dL
Chloride: 86 mg/dL
Total cholesterol: 265mg/dL
Triglycerides: 1015 mg/dL
HDL: 23 mg/dL
LDL: not calculable
Hemoglobin A1c: 15.1%
Urine with specific gravity > 1.030, glucose 3+, ketone 1+

That day we instituted an intensive in-office approach. His glucose on arrival was 596 mg/dL with other vital signs normal. His physical exam remained normal as well with the only complaints offered being fatigue and thirst. I started an intravenous (IV) line and gave him 2 liters of normal saline solution. While he was on the IV drip, he was provided a dial-a-dietician number and spoke with them to get information about how to control his new diagnosis. He received in-person education by myself and my nurse about the medication I would be prescribing him and how to check his glucose and blood pressure. He purchased these RPM products from an online retailer with instructions on how the application they were associated with works, and he was given my email address.

He received 6 units subcutaneous insulin for the hyperglycemia. Glucose and urine were repeated after the first bag of IV fluid and the second. Upon leaving the office he felt better—more hydrated and less fatigued. We repeated the labs, specifically the lipid panel and the chemistry panel, to find:

Glucose: 348 mg/dL
Sodium: 132 mg/dL
Chloride: 93 mg/dL
Total Cholesterol: 267mg/dL
Triglycerides: 689mg/dL

This patient was able to be closely monitored using telemedical follow-ups. The next day his glucose at home was 250 mg/dL and he no longer complained of thirst and fatigue. He will be closely monitored going forward and utilization of digital health will continue to be implemented.

This case demonstrates how telemedicine, telehealth, and remote patient monitoring can be utilized to keep a patient who otherwise probably would be sent to the emergency room at home. We are lucky that the practice I work for has the IV fluids available, which were vital for this patient's care. The utilization of these services allowed for close monitoring of the patient, and he expressed extreme satisfaction in the ability to maintain his care from home and avoid the emergency room, especially since this occurred during the COVID-19 pandemic.

The patient MM gave expressed verbal permission to be included in this text as a case study provided no identifying metrics were given, complying with HIPAA standards.

APPENDIX B: SAMPLE TELEMEDICAL PROTOCOLS

Protocols for Emergencies

Emergency situations can arise even from the simplest complaint. However, some complaints warrant a higher level of care than telemedicine can provide. These situations include chest pain, especially with a patient with comorbidities, abdominal pain with fever, and shortness of breath, among other concerns.

Protocols for dealing with these situations should include keeping the patient on the video chat, having a family member or staff member call 911, keeping the patient calm, and getting information together for the receiving hospital. In certain cases, such as chest pain, advising the patient take baby aspirin may be indicated. Any intervention performed should be detailed to the 911 dispatcher and any first responders that are available: EMS, police, fire/rescue.

Protocols for COVID-19 (Infectious Disease)

All practices should have an infectious disease screening tool in place. During the COVID-19 pandemic, my practice created a flow sheet to guide call center staff and receptionists in the proper means to screen patients for appropriateness of being seen in-office versus digitally. Initially, this screening tool contained travel history but that was phased out as the pandemic went on. Questions that did not change included symptoms: fever, sore throat, cough, congestion, and shortness of breath. Known exposure was also an important diagnostic factor in the telephone triage assessment for evaluation of the patient. Again, later in the pandemic this became less of a criterion as the transmission became more skewed and patients were found to contract the disease without *known* contact with an infected person.

▧ General Protocols

Overall, the patient should be screened for appropriateness. Depending on the state, a previous relationship may be required to be established prior to this visit. The call center or office receptionist should be aware of the nature of the pending telemedical visit. This will help to avoid frustration and confusion should the provider not be able to meet the needs of the patient (e.g., refill of controlled medications or a complaint that cannot meet the standard of care via telemedicine).

APPENDIX C: RECOMMENDATIONS OF BEST PRACTICES

- Have a solid knowledge of the inner workings of the chosen platform.

- All users should know the normal functions; super-rusers or practice champions should have advanced knowledge.

- Practice workflow should be implemented prior to go-live.

- Establish a back-up plan in case the primary option for digital health becomes unavailable.

- Implement appropriate protocols should emergent situations occur.

- Implement screening questions (COVID-19 or other infectious disease–related).

- All records of digital health encounters should be kept as they would for in-person evaluations.

- Be consistent in updating the practice's knowledge of rules, regulations, and laws.

- Be aware of the current climate with telemedicine.

- Have staff properly assess who is interested in digital services versus who prefers in-person evaluations.
- Be conscientious when deciding upon a self-pay rate. Should balance out cost to cover services rendered while being affordable for the patient.

APPENDIX D: SAMPLE POST-VISIT PATIENT SURVEY

1. Were you satisfied with today's care?
2. How did you find the staff treated you?
3. Did the provider make good eye contact with you?
4. Did you feel that your needs were met?
5. Did the software (Internet site, application, etc.) work as it was supposed to?
6. Would you recommend this service to friends and family?

These questions can be made to be scaled upon 1-10, yes or no, circle an appropriate answer, or any other method to collect information.

GLOSSARY

American Academy of Family Practice (AAFP): An organization that provides information and recommendations to its members and has offered several informative articles regarding telemedicine.

American Medical Association (AMA): An organization that services all physicians and has released great information about the digital health world.

American Telemedicine Association (ATA): An association made of all levels of clinicians dedicated to supporting and informing about telemedical, telehealth, and remote patient monitoring services.

Asynchronous: Synonymous with store and forward. A format of telemedicine or telehealth that involves the patient recording data and sending it to the provider at a future time.

Body mass index (BMI): A mathematical calculation of a patient's height versus weight.

Business associate agreement (BAA): A contract that specifies each party's roles and responsibilities and the consequences if these are not met.

Centers for Disease Control and Prevention (CDC): A U.S.-based organization tasked with the identification and prevention of infectious diseases. Of late they have helped with the COVID-19 pandemic and have released relevant information about digital health.

Centers for Medicare and Medicaid Services (CMS): A federal government regulatory body that offers coding, reimbursement, rules, and regulations regarding all aspects of care. They issue edicts that all practitioners, organizations, acute care hospitals, and long-term care facilities must follow if they wish to care for Medicare and Medicaid patients and bill Medicare and Medicaid.

Clinician: *See* Provider.

Coronavirus disease 2019 (COVID-19): An infectious disease that identified in China late 2019, which became a worldwide pandemic in early 2020. This disease caused a worldwide shutdown, and in the United States has infected over 40 million people, with over half a million dead as of the time of this writing.

Current Procedural Terminology (CPT): Coding for medical, surgical, and diagnostic services that allows for billing and reimbursement.

Cybersecurity: Security protocols that allow for protection of digital health services. This could be the protection of software, hardware, remote patient monitoring, or anything else regarding digital health services. This can involve built-in security, encryption, password protection, two-step verifications, and instituting protocols and policies for staff, patients, and providers to follow.

Digital health: Blanket term for providing healthcare services via electronic means.

Digital Medicine Payment Advisory Group (DMPAG): A group that functions to identify barriers to digital medicine and proposes plans on coding, payment, and insurance coverage of digital health.

Doctor of osteopathy (DO): A provider of healthcare in their chosen specialty. Usually board certified and can include primary care providers and specialists.

Durable medical equipment (DME): Medical equipment provided to help care for the patient, which can include shoes, monitoring equipment, and other supplies pertaining to the healthcare of a patient.

Electronic medical record (EMR; sometimes called electronic health records): The platform in which practices store patient information, provider and nursing notes, identification documents, laboratory and imaging results, and any other material that is part of a patient's care.

Health Insurance Portability and Accountability Act (HIPAA) of 1996: Act that required the U.S. Secretary of Health and Human Services to create protocols protecting personal health data. These can include but are not limited to demographic information, diagnostic testing, diagnosis, management, and care plans for a patient. Breach of this can result in fines, termination, or, in severe cases, incarceration.

Healthcare Common Procedure Coding System (HCPCS): A standardized method to submit claims regarding care, procedures, or management to the insurance companies, especially government-based, such as Medicare.

Hierarchical Condition Category (HCC): A system of codes based upon the ICD-10 coding system that assigns risk to a diagnostic code and along with demographic metrics allows insurance companies to associate a RAF score.

Information technologist (IT): A person or team who provides monitoring of an organization's hardware and software. These people or teams are also responsible for the cybersecurity of an organization.

Medicaid: A statewide government healthcare plan that covers indigent patients.

Medical doctor (MD): A provider of healthcare in their chosen specialty. Usually board certified and can include primary care providers and specialists.

Medicare: A government-backed healthcare plan usually provided to patients over the age of 65 or patients who are declared permanently disabled.

Nurse practitioner (NP; otherwise known as an advanced practice nurse): An advanced practice clinician who can provide independent care to a patient (depending on the state).

Physician assistant (PA): An advanced practice clinician who works with the healthcare team providing care to patients.

Point of care (POC) testing: Testing that can be completed in the office (urine pregnancy, urine dip, glucose, EKG, etc.).

Primary care provider (PCP): Clinician of any licensure who provides primary care services.

Provider: Person who provides healthcare services to a patient.

Remote patient monitoring (RPM): The ability for the patient to collect their own data and send it to the provider in real time or for future evaluation and intervention.

Risk Adjustment Factor (RAF): A scoring metric used to receive reimbursements for services provided in a full-risk network.

Store and forward: *See* Asynchronous.

Synchronous: A telemedical or telehealth approach in which a patient and provider complete their encounter via a real-time audio/video evaluation.

Telehealth: A digital means to provide health education, nurse monitoring, pharmaceutical, dietary, or other nonmedical evaluation and management.

Telemedicine: A digital approach to healthcare in which the provider (MD, DO, NP, PA) provides healthcare evaluations and management.

Vendor: The supplier of a telemedical, telehealth, or remote patient monitoring platform.

INDEX

Printed in the United States
by Baker & Taylor Publisher Services